Peripheral Nervous System

Viktor Matejčík • Zora Haviarová
Roman Kuruc

Peripheral Nervous System

Interrelationships and Variations

Springer

Viktor Matejčík
Department of Neurosurgery, Comenius University
Faculty of Medicine & University Hospital
Bratislava, Slovakia

Zora Haviarová
Institute of Anatomy, Comenius University
Faculty of Medicine
Bratislava, Slovakia

Roman Kuruc
Health Care of Surveillance Authority
Institute of Forensic Medicine
Bratislava, Slovakia

ISBN 978-3-031-73746-6 ISBN 978-3-031-73744-2 (eBook)
https://doi.org/10.1007/978-3-031-73744-2

This Springer imprint is published by the registered company Springer Nature Switzerland AG
The registered company address is: Gewerbestrasse 11, 6330 Cham, Switzerland

Preface

This work is one of the few complex documents that comprehensively evaluate the morphological and clinical aspects of the peripheral nervous system and its involvement in various pathologies. It allows a view of its topography, morphology, and peculiarities that are missing in anatomical and surgical textbooks and can complicate the solution of many pathological conditions. It attempts to comprehensively describe morphological peculiarities and their possible influence on the clinical picture. Their preoperative diagnosis is difficult, even impossible. Pictures and line drawings enrich the view of structures that have only been partially documented so far. Our observations presented in this book are based on clinical observations and systematic work on the cadavers of previously healthy people who died suddenly or violently, often as a result of car accidents. Dissection allows for an important three-dimensional view, elucidates the range of variability, and demonstrates the interdisciplinary connections between anatomy and surgical disciplines. Variations are often largely responsible for the failure of surgical treatment. They can affect the clinical picture, diagnosis, and treatment. Their recognition can minimize damage to nerve structures.

The acquired knowledge can help clarify clinical signs and symptoms in surgery or internal medicine. They may also be useful for doctors of other specialities. They can also serve as part of the undergraduate and postgraduate education of medical students and doctors or in the process of preparing other professional literature on this issue. The data presented in this publication can be useful to traumatologists, orthopaedists, spinal surgeons, neurosurgeons, plastic surgeons, neurologists, and neurophysiologists, as well as to all those who deal with or are interested in this issue.

The creation of this publication led us to develop a comprehensive view of the complexities of the peripheral nervous system, focusing on diagnosis and treatment. The scope of this monograph is not large, but it makes a significant contribution to our understanding of the diverse variations of the peripheral nervous system. It is based on the author's specific professional experience and his previous monographs on the variability of the peripheral nervous system. Note that the structure of the peripheral nervous system and its variability, due to its unpredictability, can often be associated with great complexity, sometimes as if unsolvable. The solutions cannot be written down in the form of some mathematical expression—"formula".

This work aimed to approach peripheral nerve damage not only from an anatomical point of view but also from a clinical point of view. Publications that are still in their infancy should aim for this. We believe that this book will achieve its goal and serve as a valuable reference for students and doctors seeking to extend their knowledge, as well as for compiling further professional literature on this issue.

Bratislava, Slovakia Viktor Matejčík
Bratislava, Slovakia Zora Haviarová
Bratislava, Slovakia Roman Kuruc

Acknowledgement

The authors would like to express their gratitude to Ms. Anna Francová for her help with illustrating and preparing the text of this book, Mr. Rudolf Horváth and Ms. Stanislava Horváthová for their help with the documentation, and Mr. Miroslav Rexa for proofreading the text.

Ethical Standards

The figures used in this publication depict the anatomical situation obtained through careful dissection of cadavers and within the forensic expertise with the approval of the Ethics Committee ASHC, Grösslingová 5, 812 62 Bratislava, Slovak Republic.

All studies related to the peripheral nervous system observations were conducted in accordance with all applicable standards, rules, regulations, and laws and were supervised by responsible officials.

Acknowledgement

Contents

Abbreviations

ANS	Autonomic nervous system
art.	Artery
bilat.	Bilateral
c.	Cervical
C-C	Cranio-cervical (transition)
CG	Ciliary ganglion
CN	Cranial nerve
CNS	Central nervous system
CSF	Cerebrospinal fluid
dig.	Digitorum
dors.	Dorsalis
DPN	Deep petrosal nerve
dx.	Dexter
epi.	Epineurium
ext.	External
fasc.	Fasciculus
fascc.	Fasciculi
fig.	Figure
fun.	Funiculus
GPN	Greater petrosal nerve
IHP	Inferior hypogastric plexus
inf.	Inferior
ITF	Infratemoral fossa
L	Lumbar
lat.	Lateralis
lig.	Ligamentum
LS	Lumbosacral
m.	Musculus, muscle
mm.	Musculi
n.	Nervus, nerve
NVB	Neurovascular bundle

OG	Otic ganglion
plx.	Plexus
PNS	Peripheral nervous system
post	Posterior
postfix.	Postfixed
PPF	Pterygopalatine fossa
PPG	Pterygopalatine ganglion
prefix.	Prefixed
prof.	Profundus
PSNS	Parasympathetic nervous system
r.	Ramus
rr.	Rami
seg.	Segment
sin	Sinister
SNS	Sympathetic nervous system
sulc.	Sulcus
superf.	Superficialis
symp.	Sympathetic
th.	Thoracic
tr.	Tractus
trans.	Transversus
trunc.	Truncus
v.	Vena
ventr.	Ventralis
VL	Vlákna

Part I
Morphological and Clinical Aspects of the Peripheral Nervous System and Construction and Structure of Peripheral Nerves

Chapter 1
Variability in the Peripheral Nervous System

Peripheral nerve injuries are not a marginal matter in medicine. On several pages, we tried to summarize the information related to the morphological peculiarities of the system and the possibilities of their "correction". From the patient's point of view, the consequences of injury represent long-lasting or lifetime suffering. Sometimes, even despite great effort, skill, and experience, adequate correction cannot be accomplished. Individual biological-physiological facts are applied, and we do not achieve the expected result. Success in this area is based on scientific knowledge combined with methodological experience. Knowledge of anatomy, anatomical variations, and microscopic structures is a natural requirement in the entire complex. The book is supplemented with illustrative diagrams and numerical and clinical data. Injuries and damage to peripheral nerves differ from other injuries in that their clinical course and especially clinical results are largely dependent on extremely complex processes that occur for years or decades. Information regarding the morphology of the nerves and their variations is also presented here. Illustrations direct the reader's attention to details that might be overlooked in the text but can increase the volume of clinically significant information. A picture—an illustration—is worth more than a thousand words, and we anticipate that clinical neurologists and neurosurgeons will find it a combination of the basics of anatomy, clinical neurology, and neurosurgery to update their knowledge. The publication can be an illustrative addition to the complex of neurosurgery textbooks in the framework of undergraduate education for students and physicians of postgraduate education. It will help neurologists, neurosurgeons, and doctors of other specialities to revive in their memory ideas dealing with the detailed function of nerves and muscles and the disorders of their functions that arise when individual nerve trunks are damaged. The correct and quick diagnosis of the presence of nerve injury, as well as the exact determination of its degree and nature, is of decisive importance for the outcome of the treatment. The explanation and presentation are in the dense form of symptomatology, basic facts of anatomy, physiology, semiotics, and methodology of investigation of the functions of peripheral nerves. Illustrative images and diagrams are

Z. Haviarová et al., *Peripheral Nervous System*,
https://doi.org/10.1007/978-3-031-73744-2_1

intended to support the diagnostics of traumatic lesions to nerves and their branches at different levels. We included the literature in the text only where it was necessary.

Unlike the central nervous system, injuries to the peripheral nervous system can be treated without functional deficits. However, we cannot expect a complete recovery at an older age. Injuries in the most proximal parts of the peripheral nervous system (spinal canal) lead to neuronal damage. The most serious problem is the avulsion of one or more roots from the spinal cord, which is associated with damage to the central nervous system. This kind of damage cannot be treated with a good functional result. Current treatment is therefore positive using neurotization. The most frequently used accessory nerves are intercostal nerves, nerves from the cervical plexus, phrenic nerves, or branches from the intact contralateral brachial plexus. The broken connection between the spinal cord and the periphery is compensated to some extent by means of other nerves. It is a palliative solution. Damaged spinal cord segments will be permanently disconnected from the periphery, leading to secondary changes (pain or spasticity). Peripheral nerve damage is accompanied by sensitive symptoms, muscle pain, hypotrophy, and atrophy and significantly impacts the quality of life. Limitations in normal daily activities and at work can affect the patient socially and economically. A certain variability in form, structure, and position is natural for the human body and its internal organs [1–4]. In other words, we could say that this is a tolerated natural variability. Any deviation exceeding the expected variability is usually referred to as an anomaly [5]. It is caused by different developing processes during the formation of individual structures. It can be caused by genetic, chromosomal, or environmental influences [5, 6]. Based on functional and cosmetic differences, anomalies are classified as minor and major [7, 8]. While large ones are a common cause of disease, disabilities, and death, small ones have no medical consequences [6–8]. Therefore, minor anomalies sometimes need a clear distinction from variations. Their incidence ranges from 7% to 41%, while the incidence of major anomalies is from 2% to 3% [8].

The term minor anomalies is used to describe morphological changes that can be observed from the outside (flat occiput, hypotelorism, cleft uvula, macroglossia, pigmented spots, shawl scrotum, cubitus valgus, prominent heel, etc.) [7, 8]. The presence of several minor anomalies may indicate the existence of other, much more serious defects [6, 7]. Minor anomalies should be distinguished from variations because they can be associated with major anomalies [6]. The term anomaly or malformation is used when structural changes have a negative effect on the function of the organism, as opposed to variations. However, under certain circumstances, even small, harmless variations can have a negative impact [9].

The history of anatomical variations is closely connected with the history of anatomy itself, with the history of finding and establishing images of the normal structure and composition of the human body. The ancient anatomists Galen (200–129 BC) and Vesalius (1514–1564) drew attention to individual variations. That is why we come across the expressions always, often, sometimes, rarely, and very rarely in their works. Claudius Galen was the first to describe Galen's anastomosis—the connection of nervi laryngei cum nervo laryngeo inferior, as well as venae cerebri internae and vena cerebri magna. In *De humani corporis fabrica libri septem* (1542), Andreas Vesalius described the anatomical variations of bones, muscles, and blood vessels. To understand the structure of the human body, he used dissection as the main tool. It took several centuries to establish the human body's normalities, abnormalities, and variations. This knowledge, based on the work of many anatomists, biologists, and clinicians, continues to this day in the publication of books and articles focused on anatomical variations that normally do not affect the function of the organism. Medicine needs increasingly accurate knowledge dealing with the variability of the structures of the human body to improve diagnostics and treatment. About 10% of misdiagnoses are caused by ignoring anatomical variability [6]. New and newer investigative methods have opened up space for research into anatomical variations. In our work, we focused on morphological and clinical aspects—peculiarities of the peripheral nervous system and their relationship to the surrounding structures, which often determine the success of the operation. The results of anatomical studies are necessary for a more accurate interpretation of perioperative and clinical findings. In the literature devoted to the peripheral nervous system, the question of anatomy, histology, and function is elaborated in relative detail. However, insufficient attention is paid to their mechanisms and semiotics in the aspect of tracking pathogenesis, including peripheral nerve trauma. The basis for a correct understanding of these disorders must be knowledge of the peculiarities of the structure of the plexuses and peripheral nerve trunks (Figs. 1.1 and 1.2). These peculiarities can explain the contradiction and diversity of clinical manifestations.

The presence of anastomoses indicates that each neurotome has its myotome and dermatome, but because of their complex formation, the paths of axons to the final areas of innervation are different [10].

Therefore, in the periphery, we can observe that in some cases, only one nerve supplies a certain area, and in other cases, two and sometimes three nerves participate in the innervation. In such cases, the paths of axons to the final territories are usually erratic and differ in each individual case. Knowledge about variations is important, as evidenced by the existence of many publications—usually case reports—that describe "anomalies" and "variations" of a particular nerve without a

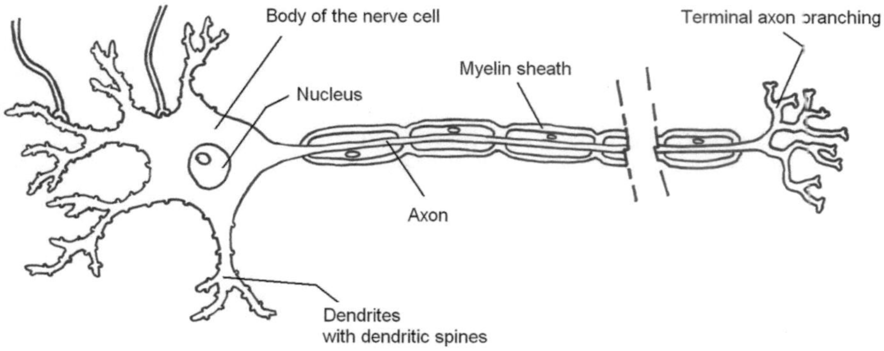

Fig. 1.1 Diagram of a nerve cell (illustrated by Ms. Anna Francová)

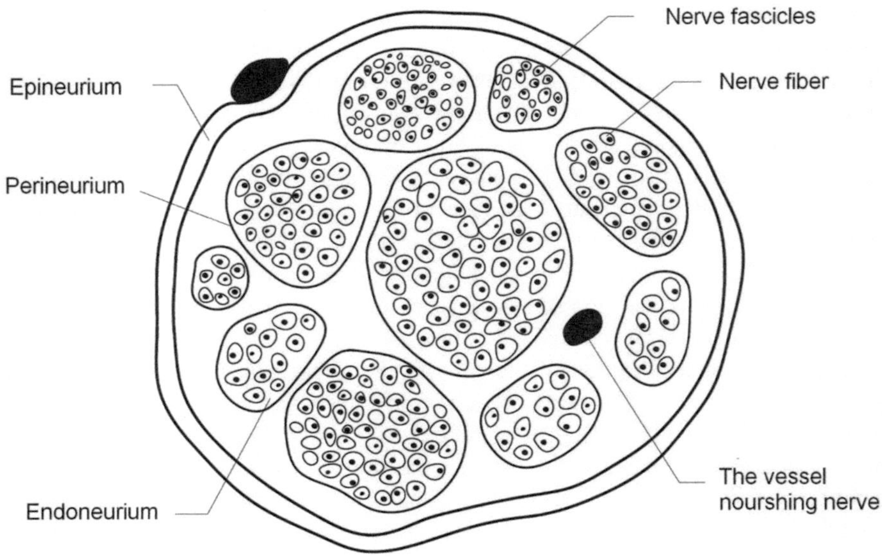

Fig. 1.2 Diagram of a peripheral nerve in cross-section (illustrated by Ms. Anna Francová)

complete analysis of the nerves as a whole in the given area. Connections between individual nerves, replacement of one nerve by another, and shift and overlapping of their innervation areas are important. Therefore, the findings, examination, and evaluation of all nerves in the given area, as well as the complex of nerves, give wide possibilities for solving several important questions.

The relationship between the CNS and the PNS is represented by the "Obersteiner-Redlich transition zone" of the brain and spinal nerves [11]. This so-called transition zone prevents the regeneration of peripheral nerves. In the transition zone, axonal growth promotes PNS tissue and inhibits CNS tissue. CN VIII is not a peripheral nerve but an outgrowth of the brain that is incapable of regeneration, just like the optic nerve (n. opticus, CN II). CN VII (facial nerve), on the other hand, is a peripheral nerve, and its "transitional zone" is almost in the brainstem. It perfectly regenerates, which is essential for the clinic. The outer border of the CNS part of the root is formed by a very irregular basement membrane of Schwann cells. The places where nerve cells pass from the PNS to the CNS part of the root are the transition between astrocytes and Schwann cells and represent a direct contact between the PNS cells of the PNS and the CNS. There is no structural boundary between the CNS and the PNS. The PNS and the CNS relationship is more of a chemical boundary based on contact inhibition that prevents one from invading the other, for example, when Schwann cells outgrow the spinal cord [12].

References

1. Fye WB. Profiles in cardiology: William Osler. Clin Cardiol. 1988;11(5):356–8.
2. Kachlík D, Varga I, Báča V, Musil V. Variant anatomy and its terminology. Medicina (Kaunas). 2020;56(12):713.
3. Bergman RA, Afifi KA, Miyauchi R. Illustrated encyclopedia of human anatomic variation. Opus III: nervous system. 2015. https://www.anatomyatlases.org/AnatomicVariants/NervousSystem/Introduction.shtml. Accessed 23 Dec 2022.
4. Šulla JI, Lukáč I, Šulla I. Syndroma cauda equinae discogenes. Košice: Univerzita Pavla Jozefa Šafárika; 2009. ISBN 978-80-7097-769-9.
5. Arey LB. Development anatomy. Philadelphia and London: W.B. Saunders Company; 1940.
6. Holmes LB. Current concepts in genetics. Congenital malformations. N Engl J Med. 1976;295(4):204–7.
7. Marden PM, Smith DW, McDonald MJ. Congenital anomalies in the newborn infant, including minor variations. J Pediatr. 1964;64:357–71.
8. Stevenson RE, Hall JG. Terminology, 1. In: Stevenson RE, Hall JG and Goodman RM (eds.). Human malformations and related anomalies. Oxford University Press, London. 1993, 21-30.
9. Lippert H, Pabst R. Arterial variations in man classification and frequency. München: J.F. Bergman Verlag; 1985.
10. Urbanowitz Z. Connections between the lumbal and sacral plexus in man. Folia Morphol (Warsz). 1981;40(3):271–9.
11. Obersteiner H, Redlich E. Uber wesen und Patogenese der Tabischen Hinterstrangs Degeneration. ARB Neurol Inst Univ Wien. 1894;1-3:158–72.
12. Zvěřina E, Chovanec M, Betka J. Rekonštrukční operace lícního nervu v zadní jáme a v mostovomozečkového koutu. In: Vachata P, Sameš M, et al., editors. Lícní nerv. Mladá: Fronta; 2016. p. 141–59. ISBN 978-80-204-3252-0.

Chapter 2
Definition of the Terms About the Peripheral Nervous System

Peripheral nerves connect the central nervous system with peripheral receptors and executive organs through a system of afferent and efferent sensory, motor, and autonomic fibres. They are of different thicknesses and can be myelinated or unmyelinated. The peripheral nerve transmits information in the form of nerve impulses. The basic nerve unit is the axon—the protrusion of the nerve cell ensuring axoplasmic transport (Fig. 1.1). Several nerve fibres (axons) are connected in a bundle—a fascicle. Inside the bundle between the nerve fibres is a connective tissue—endoneurium. It contains mucopolysaccharides, collagen, reticulin, cells (fibroblasts, macrophages), and blood vessels. Each fascicle, which contains an average of 10,000 axons, has an outer covering—perineurium (Fig. 1.2). The perineurium forms the morphological unit of the fascicle. It is composed of an inner layer of scaly cells and an outer layer of collagen fibres. It also contains vessels connecting the endoneurial and epineural vascular networks. Between the fascicles, there is connective tissue—the internal epineurium.

The microcirculation for each fascicle is localized in the sparse connective tissue of the epineurium that surrounds it. The internal circulation is supplied through the mesoneurium. The mesoneurium carries blood vessels to the nerve. The entire nerve is surrounded by an external epineurium, which connects the nerve to the surrounding structures through the mesoneurium. The epineurium forms a collagen-elastic matrix in fibroblasts, mastoid cells, and blood vessels.

The endoneurium, perineurium, and epineurium form the connective tissue of the peripheral nerve, which not only connects but also isolates and separates one part of the nerve from another. The amount of connective tissue in a nerve depends on the type of nerve and its level.

Each fascicle in the nerve can move forward and backward inside it with the help of the thin connective tissue that covers it. This allows independent movement around adjacent fascicles and the outer surface of the nerve, region of the plexus roots, trunks, fascicles, and terminal branches of the brachial and lumbosacral plexus around the surrounding structures. A large amount of sparse connective

Z. Haviarová et al., *Peripheral Nervous System*,
https://doi.org/10.1007/978-3-031-73744-2_2

tissue ensures the mobility of the fascicles among themselves and of the nerve with its surroundings [1–5]. In areas such as the shoulder, elbow, and wrist, where great mobility of the nerve is required, the mesoneurium is longer and more complex and contains more vessels. When the tension on the nerve relaxes during flexion in the joint, the blood vessels undulate and contract like an accordion. As the tension increases during movement, the vessels in the mesoneurium align and adapt to the position of the nerve. The mesoneurium and its vessels appear to be responsible for the retraction of the nerve endings when it is cut, as evidenced by the retraction of the nerve after its interruption.

In the event of a cutting injury, each fascicle can move forward or backward. This explains why some fascicles give an image with characteristic kinks. The surrounding supporting tissue that keeps them upright and stretched is damaged and therefore unable to perform its role. These changes are the result of the formation of connective tissue, the longer the time passes from the injury to the operation. A larger amount of connective tissue reduces the chance of excellent adjustment of its functions. Peripheral nerves have considerable strength and elasticity due to the perineurium, which maintains the integrity of the nerve roots under tension.

The clinical symptomatology of peripheral nerve damage consists of movement or sensitivity disorders and vascular or motor disorders of nerve trunk functions. The extent of impairment depends on the level of nerve damage. The neurological picture of the lesion can be complicated by damage to muscles, bones, and blood vessels. Damage to the muscle leads to its fibrotization, shortening of the tendons, fusion with the surrounding tissues, and thus also subsequent limited movement of the joints.

Contractures and restrictions of movement in the joints impede a perfect examination of the nerve's function. Nerve irritation can lead to an increase in muscle tone, and the limb can be in a non-physiological position.

Damage to vessels inside or outside the nerve also leads to a decrease in the function of nerves that are not directly damaged by the trauma, which significantly complicates clinical symptomatology. Bleeding itself can be the cause of significant pain due to irritation of the sympathetic fibres of blood vessels. Soreness can prevent active movement of that group of muscles whose innervation is not disturbed. Great problems in determining paresis or plegia of the corresponding muscles can be caused by the presence of nerve anastomoses and variations when the function of damaged muscles is replaced by neighbouring ones. Another important symptom of nerve damage is sensitivity disorders. They are manifested by several signs that may indicate the degree of nerve damage and the course of regeneration. Different types of sensitivity have different thresholds for nerve damage and regeneration. Impairment of sensitivity due to nerve damage can be manifested in the form of pain or paresthesia. Pain can appear from the moment of injury, or it can appear over time.

It can be related to nerve irritation, the formation of fibrotic changes or neuroma, or an inflammatory process. Projection pain when compressing the nerve below the site of injury indicates the absence of anatomical disruption of the nerve. In case of its interruption, the pain does not appear. The appearance of pain during later examinations can be an early sign of regeneration. It should be noted that there are no absolute criteria for anatomical interruption of the nerve. Manifestations of nerve irritation also include the clinical picture known as causalgia. It occurs when a nerve is partially damaged. It can be associated with irritation of sympathetic fibres. The frequent occurrence of causalgia observed in the case of a lesion of the median nerve (n. medianus) and tibial nerve (n. tibialis) is explained by the presence of many sympathetic fibres. Another important symptom of peripheral nerve damage is the presence of vasomotor, secretory, and trophic disorders. Vasomotor disorders in the case of nerve interruption are manifested by cyanosis, which is accentuated by cooling. Its boundaries correspond to the territory of the nerve and depend on the paralysis of vasoconstrictors. In cases of nerve irritation, reddening of the skin and a feeling of heat or burning sensation are observed, which tend to be particularly pronounced in causalgia. A combination of cyanosis and reddening of the skin often occurs. Significant swelling of the limbs can be observed due to a change in blood vessel tone. Along with vasomotor changes in the innervation of the injured nerve, secretion disturbances such as hyperhidrosis or anhidrosis, as well as trophic disorders, can be observed. In case of complete interruption of the nerve, the skin is thin, hair growth is absent, nails become thinner, and their growth slows down. Nerve irritation can be manifested by peeling of the skin, hyperkeratosis, hypertrichosis, accelerated growth, and thickening of the nails. Trophic influences are manifested in the development of muscle atrophy and impaired wound healing. Fibrous thickenings are sometimes formed in the tendons and fibrous sheaths, which lead to the development of contractures. Decalcification or osteoporosis is often observed on X-ray examination. Recognition of a nerve lesion becomes reliable when motor, sensory, reflex, secretory, and/or trophic changes occur simultaneously.

The diversity and variability of clinical manifestations of nerve injury in different people are because the same nerve contains different numbers of myelinated and unmyelinated fibres. The largest number of autonomic nerve fibres is mainly in the median nerve and tibial nerve. Atypical localization of the difficulties is explained by the presence of anastomoses of the damaged nerve with surrounding ones. It occurs when nerve conduction is partially impaired, and the cause can be scar tissue, intraneural neuromas, and fibrous changes. The work aims to point out the anatomical variations of the peripheral nervous system and their participation in the clinic. In the literature available to us, we have come across only a few works devoted to this issue. We did not find works aimed at the bilateral detection of anatomical deviations in the formation of the entire peripheral nervous system and their possible impact on the clinic.

Many variations in the formation of the cervical, brachial, and lumbosacral plexus are, in addition to atypical clinical and electromyographic findings, a source of diagnostic confusion. It is important to understand which nerve functions are transmitted in individual parts of the plexus. At the same time, it should be considered that due to the presence of various connections between the roots of the plexus, the innervation of the muscles and the clinical symptomatology may change. In the prefixed type, the nerve roots receive more fibres from more cranial spinal nerves. Damage to high spinal roots or nerves is accompanied by a much more widespread lesion in the periphery than that is caused by the same type of injury—damage in the postfixed type [6–13]. It is hard to imagine that differences in the structure of the nervous system would not be reflected in pain irradiation. A certain agreement of anatomical differences with differences in the clinical picture is known and observed in the spinal nerve system, where there are greater opportunities for objective observation than in the autonomic nervous system (see also Part VI, Chap. 18 Figs. 18.48 and 18.49).

References

1. Arey LB. Development anatomy. Philadelphia and London: W.B. Saunders Company; 1940.
2. Zvěřina E, Stejskal L. Poranění periférních nervů. Praha: Avicenum; 1979. p. 303.
3. Wiliams PL. Nervous system in Gray's anatomy. 38th ed. New York: Churchill Livingstone; 1995. p. 1267–72.
4. Tubbs RS, Shoja MM. Loukas M (Eds.). Bergman's comprehensive encyclopedia of human anatomic variation. Hoboken, NJ: John Wiley & Sons; 2016.
5. Rouviére H, Delmas A. Anatomie humaine. Descriptive, topographique et fonctionelle. 15th ed. Paris: Masson; 2002. p. 1–784. ISBN 9782294003929.
6. Haninec P, Kaiser R. Operační léčba poranění plexus brachialis. ČSl Neurol Neurochir. 2011;74/107(5):619–30.
7. Bergman RA, Thompson SA, Afifi AK, Saddeh FA. Compendium of human anatomical variations. Baltimore: Urban and Schwarzenburg; 1988. p. 138–9.
8. Hauck EF, Wittkowski W, Bothe HW. Intradural microanatomy of the nerve roots S1-S5 at their origin from the conus medullaris. J Neurosurg Spine. 2008;9(2):207–12.
9. Moore KL. Clinically oriented anatomy. 2nd Baltimore, Williams & Wilkins; 1985, 626–793.
10. Balik V, Šulla I. Autonomic Dysreflexia following spinal cord injury. Asian J Neurosurg. 2022;17(2):165–72.
11. Baader B, Herrmann M. Topography of the pelvic autonomic nervous system and its potential impact on surgical intervention in the pelvis. Clin Anat. 2003;16(2):119–30.
12. Moore KL, Dalley AL. Clinically oriented anatomy II. 5th ed. Baltimore, MD: Williams; 2006. p. 321.
13. Hulín I, et al. Patofyziológia. Faber; 1998. p. 1141.

Part II
The Spinal Nerves, The Autonomic Nervous System and the Followed Material

Chapter 3
Differences in the Structure of the Autonomic Nervous System and the Structure of the Followed Material

We completely examined 243 human cadavers (ages ranging from 30–86 years old), without any congenital or acquired anomalies, cancer, orthopaedic deformities, and spinal or abdominal operations within 24 h of death. In 50 corpses, the extradural cervicobrachial plexus and lumbosacral plexus were revealed. Intraspinal variations of peripheral nerves were revealed in 43 corpses and intracranial intradural cranial nerves in 60 cases, and the autonomic nervous system was revealed in 20 corpses. In 20 cases, intracranial variations of the autonomic ganglia of the cranial nerves were revealed.

In the cervical region, we defined the level of the vertebrae by manual subtraction from the C-C transition and the roots from the C2 root. In the prefixed type, the C4 root participated in the formation of the brachial plexus in two cases (4%). In the postfixed type, roots T1 and T2 participated in one case (2%). In such cases, the T1 root has the number of fibres normally carried by the C8 root, and the contribution of the T2 root to the plexus may be greater. In the lumbosacral region, the roots were defined based on their participation in the formation of plexuses. In the prefixed type, the anterior branch of the L4 root was thicker or as thick as the L5, S1, and S2 roots, i.e., the thicker lumbosacral trunk (truncus lumbosacralis) was present. In the postfixed type, the junction from the L4 root to the L5 root was thin, and the anterior roots S3, S4, and S5 were more distinctive.

Differences in the Structure of the Autonomic Nervous System

In 20 cadavers, the peripheral autonomic nervous system was dissected bilaterally, and the body was in the supine position. Subsequently, a "scarf" skin incision was made on both sides along the clavicle to its lateral part. We relocated the skin and subcutaneous tissue upwards. The clavicles were separated from the sternal manubrium, the ribs were cut in the mid-axillary line, and the anterior chest wall was

Z. Haviarová et al., *Peripheral Nervous System*, https://doi.org/10.1007/978-3-031-73744-2_3

removed. First, we dissected the vagus nerve, sympathetic trunk, spinal nerves with their branches, and the phrenic nerve. In cadavers of older people, the elasticity of the nerves and their strength were significantly reduced. After examination and removal of the lungs and mediastinal contents, the parietal pleura was carefully retracted to expose the thoracic prevertebral sympathetic chains, ganglia, and the thoracic splanchnic nerves, and most of the diaphragm was removed except for areas that were firmly attached to the posterior thoracic wall. After identifying the thoracic sympathetic ganglia, the sympathetic chain, and the thoracic splanchnic nerves, the connections between the ganglia and the thoracic splanchnic nerves were traced. Access to the nervous structures of the abdominal cavity, including the autonomic nervous system, was gained through a longitudinal incision in the midline from the xiphoid process to the symphysis, bypassing the umbilicus. An incision was made through the linea alba and the anterior wall of the peritoneal sac, exposing the peritoneal cavity. An oblique incision along the mesentery was made from the suspensory muscle of the duodenum toward the cecum. Ascending and descending colons were mobilized by severing the right and left paracolic radix of the mesentery, and the sigmoid colon was separated from the rectum. The intestines, pancreas, and remaining posterior parietal peritoneum were swept up to expose the infrarenal retroperitoneum. After the examination and removal of the organs of the abdominal cavity, the celiac plexus became clearly visible in its entirety. Increased attention was paid to the renal vessels, urethra, inferior mesenteric and gonadal vessels, and plexuses. Dissection of the aortic plexus was complete after identification of the lumbar splanchnic nerves in the interaortocaval fat. The right splanchnic nerves were followed posteriorly to locate the right sympathetic chain and anteriorly to isolate the preaortic nerves—aortic plexus. Dissection of the left sympathetic chain and left lumbar splanchnic nerves followed, providing a basis for examination of each preaortic nerve to distinguish intermesenteric nerves from the aortic plexus from the nerves running within the mesenteric plexus. In the pelvic part, we dissected the superior and inferior hypogastric plexus, rectal plexus, urinary bladder, and communications of the sympathetic trunk. After partial retroperitoneal clarification of the pelvic splanchnic nerves entering the pelvic plexus from the anterior, lateral, and laterocaudal approaches, the pelvic organs were removed by separating the peritoneum from the symphysis. Semicircular movements of the fingers of both hands gradually separated the viscera of the small pelvis from its wall on the right, left, and back, until the fingers of both hands touched behind the rectum. We strained the entire complex cranially and severed the ureter in men below the prostate and in women below the bladder, as well as the vagina and rectum. We separated the rectum from the frontal surface of the sacrum with a pull or with a sharp knife, and we cut through the peritoneum on both sides and removed the entire complex of viscera out of the small pelvis. Subsequently, we dissected the pelvic plexus and nerve structures innervating the bladder, prostate, and seminal vesicles lying laterally, cranially, and dorsally from the prostate between the bladder and the rectum. We dilated the inguinal canal with two fingers up to the middle of the scrotum. By pressing on the lower pole of the scrotum, we pushed the testis and epididymis upwards and visualized the spermatic plexus (plexus spermaticus) and deferential plexus (plexus deferentialis). The fascial structures covering the sacral nerve roots were excised. The parasympathetic nerve roots were identified after their origin from the S2–S4 anterior nerve roots and dissected along their course forward to their exit at the lateral border of the rectum.

Importance of Data on Extreme Types of the Autonomic Nervous System

The complexity and significant instability of the clinical picture of the same disease in different individuals are also due to the structure of the peripheral part of the autonomic nervous system [1–6]. It is difficult to imagine that differences in the structure of the autonomic nervous system would not be reflected in pain irradiation. Anatomical data also show that only in one-third of cases, there are direct anatomical paths of pain propagation. The irritation coming from the internal organs spreads to the corresponding segments of the spinal cord and subsequently manifests itself on the periphery as “defense musculaire”. Anatomical differences in junctions between the autonomic and spinal systems are important. In cases where the ganglia in the sympathetic trunk (truncus sympathicus) are distributed segmentally and each ganglion has communicating branches (rr. communicantes) with the corresponding spinal nerve, it can be clearly assumed that the irritation emanating from the internal organs will spread to the nearest given organ to the segment/segments in the area of “defense” extension and will largely correspond to the territory of the actual organ. In other cases, in a concentration of ganglionic masses, when one ganglion is connected with several spinal nerves, the irritation will spread to several segments, sometimes seemingly unrelated to the diseased organ. In these cases, one can expect that the area of increased muscle tension will spread beyond the distribution of the pathological process. There is not a single organ in the abdominal cavity whose disease would not be accompanied by pain in the celiac region, at least to some degree. This condition is explained by the fact that the celiac plexus (which is the “centre” of pain) is connected with the plexuses of other organs. In those cases where the ganglion masses in the prevertebral section are scattered, when a large number of small ganglia are present (as if a large number of separate local “centres” of pain), pain in the region of the celiac plexus may not be as precisely localized as in a distinct concentration (in the presence of two, rarely of three large ganglia forming a plexus). At the beginning of every pathological process in the internal organs, there are painful sensations in the boundaries of the celiac plexus. They sometimes spread very quickly, sometimes slowly, to other areas, via the path of pain irradiation. Their localization points are different, and it is more difficult to determine their specificity for a particular organ. This diversity from the point of view of irradiation can be explained by differences in the structure of the celiac plexus. Irritation of the celiac plexus caused by a painful condition can spread to different areas of the body, which often do not have a segmental connection with the actual organ. The figures show the spread of pain depending on the type of formation of the greater splanchnic nerve (n. splanchnicus major), with "high" type (Fig. 3.1) and with "low" type of formation (Figs. 3.2, 3.3, 3.4).

Figure 3.3 shows the possible path of pain propagation in a pathological condition—most often in acute liver damage and inflammation of the gall bladder or bile ducts. Here, the pain reaches the celiac plexus (1) from the point of origin, followed by the branches forming the diaphragmatic plexus (2), through which is often possible to observe—the accumulation of ganglion cells (3). Here, the phrenic nerve (n. phrenicus) divides into final branches, and after the trunk of the last one (4) through the cervical plexus (plexus cervicalis) (C2, C3, C4), they penetrate the segments of the spinal cord, which are the source of the supraclavicular nerves (5). Since the described path does not always exist (connections of the phrenic nerve with the celiac plexus are missing in 1/3–2/3 of the cases), this results in the instability of pain irradiation to the supraclavicular area and the right shoulder (instability of the connections between the phrenic nerve and the celiac plexus). The rarely observed radiation of pain in diseases of the biliary tract to the left arm is explained by the great rarity of connections between the left phrenic nerve (n. phrenicus) and the celiac plexus. This is confirmed by the discovery of zones of hyperesthesia in the

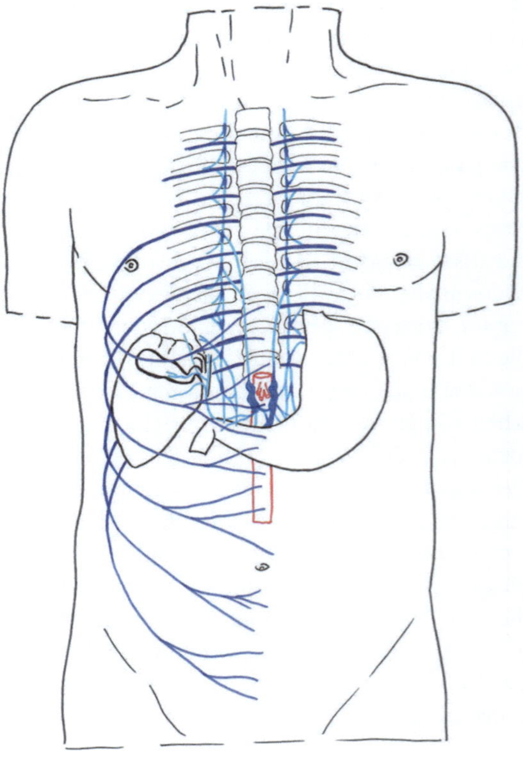

Fig. 3.1 Irradiation of pain in diseases of the liver or bile ducts with a low type of formation of the greater splanchnic nerve (n. splanchnicus major) (illustrated by Ms. Anna Francová)

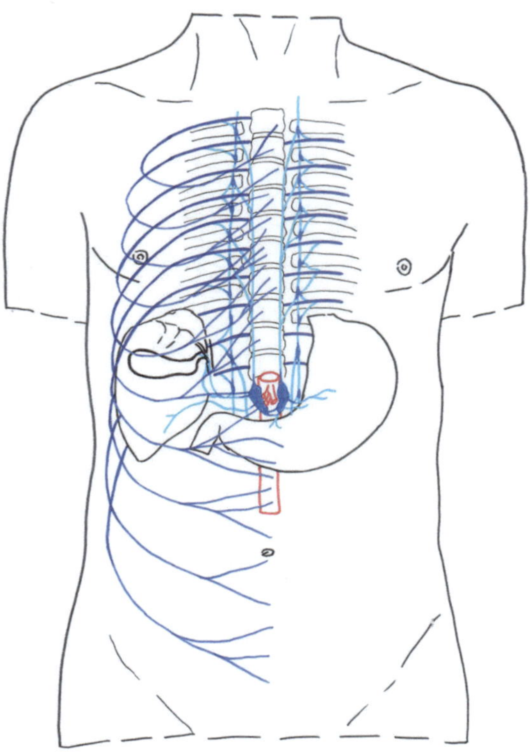

Fig. 3.2 Irradiation of pain from the celiac plexus in case of a high type of formation of the greater splanchnic nerve (n. splanchnicus major) (illustrated by Ms. Anna Francová)

shoulder area when the phrenic nerve branches are irritated in case of a pathological process under the dome of the diaphragm (adrenal tumours, liver disease). Figure 3.4 shows the zones of the spread of hyperesthesia in tumours of the adrenal glands (from the left). Here, the pain arises at the borders of the diaphragm (the result of its compression) and spreads along the trunk of the phrenic nerves (nn. phrenici) (1) to the corresponding segment of the spinal cord and from there through the supraclavicular nerves (nn. supraclaviculares) (2) reaching the clavicle and the shoulder. Significant hyperesthesia can sometimes appear in the mentioned area (3). Pain in the shoulder area is observed following gastric, duodenal, or intestinal perforation when the spilt collection reaches the diaphragm and irritates the endings of the phrenic nerves (nn. phrenici) (see also Part VI. Chap. 18: Figs. 18.48 and 18.49).

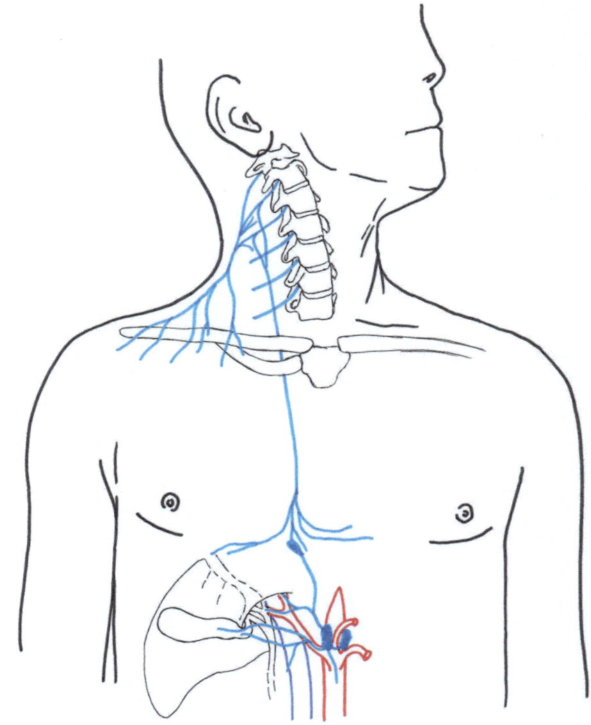

Fig. 3.3 Possible paths of pain propagation in liver and biliary tract involvement (illustrated by Ms. Anna Francová)

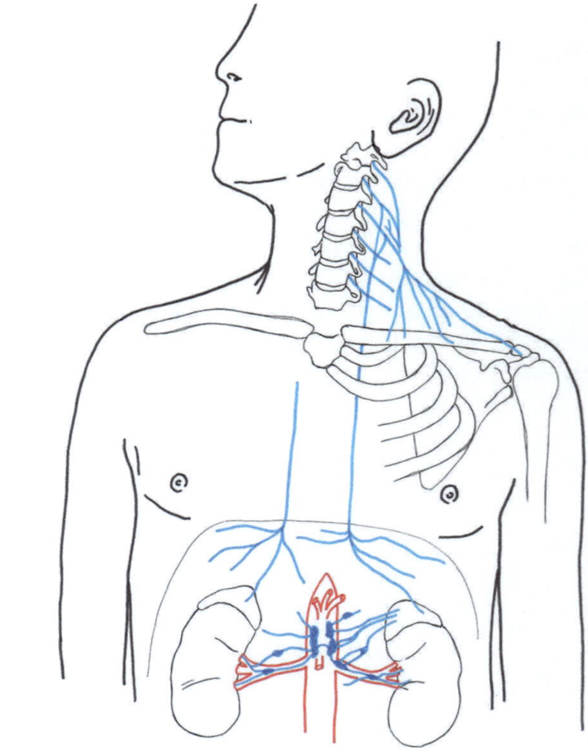

Fig. 3.4 Zones of pain propagation in adrenal tumours (from left) (illustrated by Ms. Anna Francová)

References

1. Gandhi KR, Verma VK, Chavan SK, Joshi SD, Joshi SS. The morphology of lumbar sympathetic trunk in humans: a cadaveric study. Folia Morphol (Warsz). 2013;72(3):217–22.
2. Loukas M, Klaassen Z, Merbs W, Tubbs RS, Gielecki J, Zurada A. A review of the thoracic splanchnic nerves and celiac ganglia. Clin Anat. 2010;23(5):512–22.
3. Ward EM, Rorie DK, Nauss LA, Bahn RC. The celiac ganglia in man: normal anatomic variations. Anesth Analg. 1979;58(6):461–5.
4. Karemaker JM. An introduction into autonomic nervous function. Physiol Meas. 2017;38(5):R89–R118.
5. Yang HJ, Gil YC, Lee WJ, Kim TJ, Lee HY. Anatomy of thoracic splanchnic nerves for surgical resection. Clin Anat. 2008;21(2):171–7.
6. Edwards LF, Baker RC. Variations in the formation of the splanchnic nerves in man. Anat Rec. 1940;77(3):335–42.

Chapter 4
Differences in the Structure of the Brachial Plexus

We focused our work concerning the brachial plexus on determining the topography of anatomical deviations from its nerve roots to the terminal branches. We studied 50 cadavers, in all of which the brachial plexuses were visualized bilaterally. The body was in a supine position with the limb slightly extended. The skin incision was made from the upper third of the lateral side of the sternocleidomastoid muscle (m. sternocleidomastoideus) to the medial third of the clavicle and from there along the clavicle to its lateral end and then through the deltoid-pectoral groove to the inner surface of the shoulder to its lower third. We set aside the skin and subcutaneous tissue. First, we dealt with the supraclavicular part of the plexus. We exposed the spinal nerves at the intraforaminal level up to the edge of the dura by resection of the ends of the transverse processes (processus transversi). When it was necessary to isolate the upper plexus, the C7 spinal root, and the C7 root as the middle trunk or C8 and T1 of the lower trunk, we removed the insertion of the anterior scalene muscle (m. scalenus anterior) to the frontal tubercles or cut part of the anterior scalene muscle (m. scalenus anterior). Space of the long thoracic nerve (n. thoracicus longus) was found by lifting the C6 root forward. After dissecting the trunks and their branches, the next phase followed. It consisted of the separation of the pectoralis major muscle (m. pectoralis major) in the range of 2–3 cm from the clavicle and the clavicle from the medial to its lateral third. At this stage, the clavicle-pectoral aponeurosis, subclavius muscle (m. subclavius), and pectoralis minor muscle (m. pectoralis minor) were separated, which made it possible to reveal the lower trunk and medial fascicle. On the section in the front covered by the pectoralis minor muscle, the nerve roots of the plexus were located close to each other and extended around the artery. Partial cutting of the pectoralis minor and major muscles finally made it possible to see the infraclavicular part of the brachial plexus and all pectoral nerves as well as the terminal nerves in their entirety. For the more proximal dissection, we initially exposed the lateral fascicle, which was fixed by connective tissue fibres to the fascia of the subclavius muscle. The medial fascicle is located inward from the lateral one and deeper. By dissection near it, we located the posterior

Z. Haviarová et al., *Peripheral Nervous System*,
https://doi.org/10.1007/978-3-031-73744-2_4

fascicle. At the level of the origin of the coracobrachialis branches from the lateral fascicle, there is a bifurcation of the posterior fascicle into the radial nerve (n. radialis) and axillary nerve (n. axillaris). By deeper preparation down to the lower border of the projection of the pectoralis minor muscle, we exposed the median nerve. When working from the bottom up, dissection around the proximal part of the median nerve led to the lateral and medial roots of the fork of the median nerve.

We used the distance level of the axillary nerve (n. axillaris) from the posterior fascicle as a reference point. Proximally to this level were the fascicles and the distal nerves that originate from them. The creation of fascicles was carried out, as a rule, not higher than the level of the projection of the lower edge of the clavicle. By the term "root", we define a network, not a spinal root, that is, the pretrunkal part of the plexus, including the segment of the spinal nerve up to the plexus trunk.

Differences in the Structure and Lesions of the Brachial Plexus at the Level of the Plexus Nerve Roots

The anterior branches of C5–C8 and partially T1 participate in the formation of the brachial plexus.

However, we can often see that the C4 and T2 roots also can participate in the formation of the brachial plexus.

In some cases (Fig. 4.1), the roots of C5–T2 participate in the formation of the plexus, too. While the T2 root [1] is relatively thin, the anastomoses with the cervical plexus are in the C4–C5 range [2].

In other cases (Fig. 4.2), the roots of C4–T1 participate in forming the brachial plexus.

We also find another type of formation (Fig. 4.3).

When comparing the given images, it can be seen that in one case, the plexus is displaced in the caudal direction and, in the other case, in the cranial direction. Moreover, segments C4 and sometimes C3 participate in its formation (Fig. 4.2).

In the first case, the T2 segment participates in the formation of the plexus (Fig. 4.1). These shifts explain the differences that are observed in the clinical presentation of the brachial plexus lesions.

In the prefixed type, the nerve roots receive more fibres from higher nerves [1, 2]. The C4 root can make a major contribution to the suprascapular nerve or even the axillary nerve. The radial nerve (n. radialis) receives more C5 fibres, and the same is observed about the musculocutaneous nerve (n. musculocutaneus) and others (all the found results are presented in Table 4.1).

In the first case, damage to the C5 root can be accompanied by plegia not only of the deltoid muscle (m. deltoid), biceps brachii muscle (m. biceps brachii), and brachialis muscle (m. brachialis), but also plegia of the wrist extensors such as m. brachioradialis, m. supinator, and m. pronator teres. The same damage to the C5 root in cases of caudal placement of the plexus may not affect the function of the forearm muscles at all, or the brachialis muscle and biceps brachii muscles can be

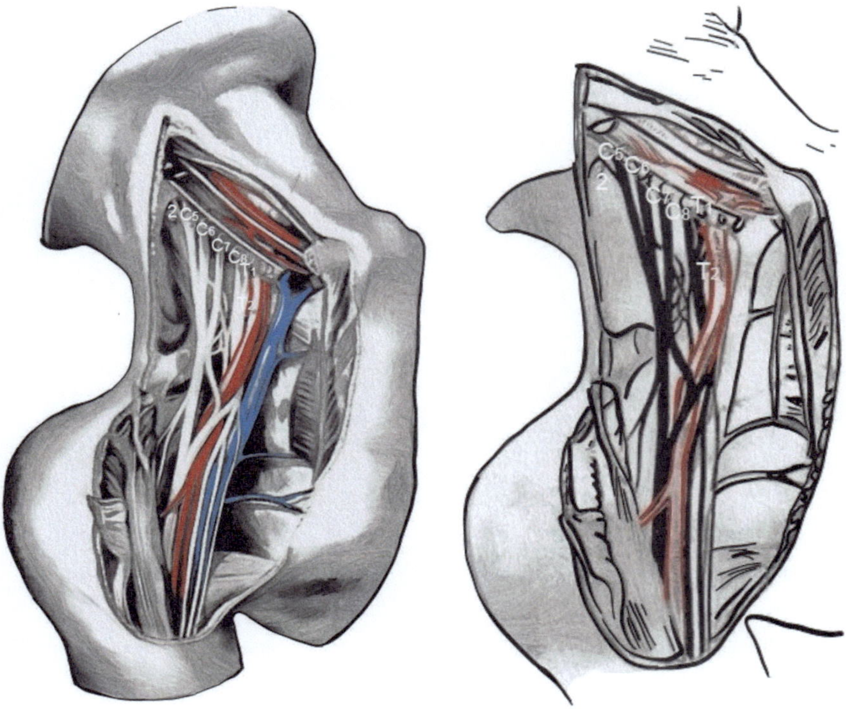

Fig. 4.1 The C5–T2 roots participate in the formation of the brachial plexus. While the T2 root is relatively thin, the anastomoses of the cervical plexus are in the C4–C5 range [2] (illustrated by Ms. Anna Francová)

only partially affected. Damage to high-lying nerves or nerve trunks (such as the superior trunk) is accompanied by a much more widespread plegia than is caused by the same damage in the postfixed type.

In the postfixed type [1, 2], the T1 root may have the number of fibres normally carried in the C8 root, and the contribution of T2 to the plexus may be greater. The C7 root provides a predominant innervation of the limb and participates to a greater or lesser extent in the formation of all nerve trunks of the upper limb. In rare cases of a lesion, we observe a rather diffuse loss of function, without complete anaesthesia or paralysis of any significant muscle group. The eighth cervical nerve participates in the innervation of the extensors of the fingers and thumb. The first thoracic nerve does the same to a lesser extent and is also partially involved in the innervation of the triceps brachii muscle (m. triceps brachii).

We did not observe the simultaneous participation of the C4 and T2 roots in the formation of the brachial plexus. The roots that formed the plexus generally passed through the gap between the anterior and middle scalene muscles (m. scalenus anterior et medius), but in one case, the C5 root and, in another one, both the C5 and C6 roots passed through the anterior scalene muscle. In five cases, only part of the C5

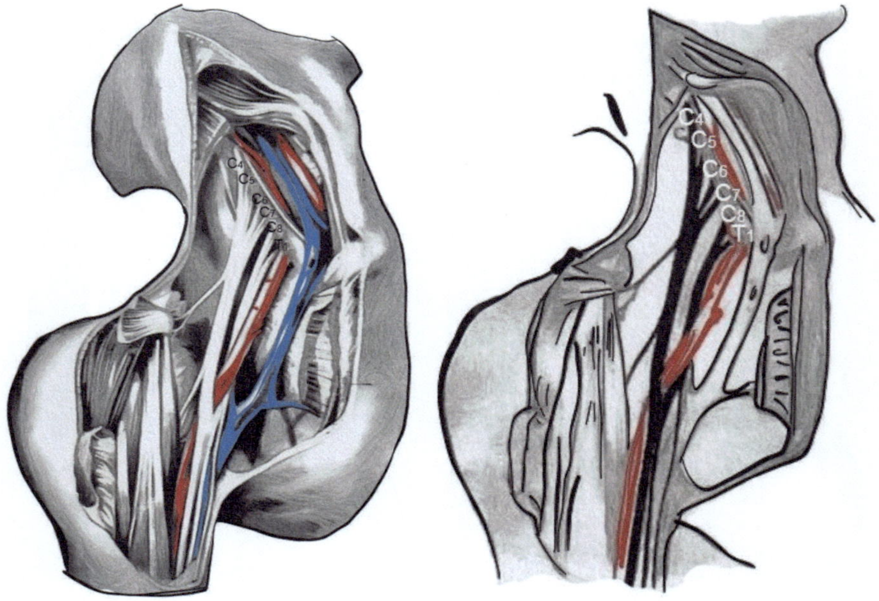

Fig. 4.2 The roots C4 and sometimes C3 participate in the formation of the brachial plexus (illustrated by Ms. Anna Francová)

root was involved in the formation of the brachial plexus, and the other part was connected to the C4 root. The phrenic nerve was in one cadaver connected to the C5 root by one branch and in two corpses by several branches. The most proximal branch of the C5 root is the dorsalis scapulae nerve (n. dorsalis scapulae). In 4 cases, it was observed to arise from the underside of the C6 root. The long thoracic nerve (n. thoracicus longus) was formed from contributions from C5 in all cases; in 16 cases (32%) from C5, C6, and C7; and in four cases from C4, C5, and C6. Mostly, it originated only from C5 and C6 roots—in 35 cases (70%). The largest trunk was always from the C6 root.

Of the three branches of the nerve roots, two appear to be clinically important—the long thoracic nerve (n. thoracicus longus) and the dorsal scapular nerve (n. dorsalis scapulae). If the muscles innervated by these nerves are not functional, a proximal plexus root injury or spinal cord avulsion is suspected. On the other hand, if the muscles innervated by these nerves are functional (even if no other muscles are functional), the preservation of the proximal nerve fibres is assumed. They can be identified during surgery and used in the reconstruction of the brachial plexus. The root supply of the pectoralis major muscle (m. pectoralis major) (C5–T1) is a reduced image of the state of the entire brachial plexus. The clavicular part is supplied from the roots of C5 and C6, the sternal part from C7, and the abdominal part from C8–T1 via the pectoral nerves. It clinically corresponds to the upper, middle, and lower types of brachial plexus lesions. This may be of importance in locating

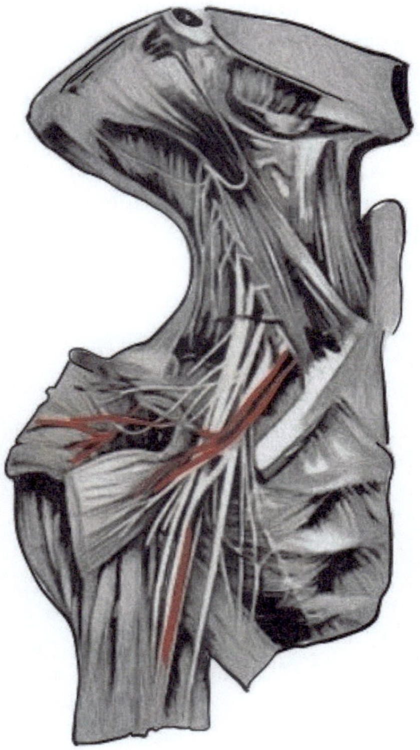

Fig. 4.3 Another type of formation (illustrated by Ms. Anna Francová)

Table 4.1 Variations of the brachial plexus at the level of trunk roots

Plexus brachialis	SIN.	DX.	Bilat.
C5 and C6 roots are divided into anterior and posterior branch	2		
C7 root is thin without the anterior branch	1		1
C7 root issues a branch toward the C8 root	1		1
C8 root issues two branches toward the posterior fascicle of the middle trunk	1		1
C8 divides into two branches, the anterior toward the anterior division of the superior trunk, the posterior joins T1			1
C8 root joins the anterior branch of C6 via two branches	1		
C8 branches join the lateral and posterior fascicle	1		
T1 root thicker than C8	2	1	
Total	**9**	**1**	**4**

SIN. sinister, *DX.* dexter, *Bilat.* bilateral

lesions at the level of fascicles. Even if the C5, C6, C7, and C8 nerves are interrupted, the injured person may still be able to move the shoulder. The movement can be caused by the function of the accessory nerve (CN XI, n. accesorius) and cervical plexus. The biceps brachii muscle can restore its function in some cases even with a complete type of plexus injury with root avulsion. Roots C3 and C4 and phrenic nerve are also involved in innervation. Knowledge of anatomical variations can contribute to the explanation of incomprehensible clinical symptoms. We found anatomical deviations in the formation of the axillary nerve (n. axillaris)—as a continuation of the posterior branch of the upper trunk. The anatomical arrangement of the brachial plexus is complex, and when developing the clinical picture, its diagnosis, and surgical treatment, individual specific variants must be considered. It will help to prevent surprises from certain operative findings. (Figs. 4.4, 4.5, 4.6) (see also Part VI, Chap. 18: Figs. 18.1–18.6).

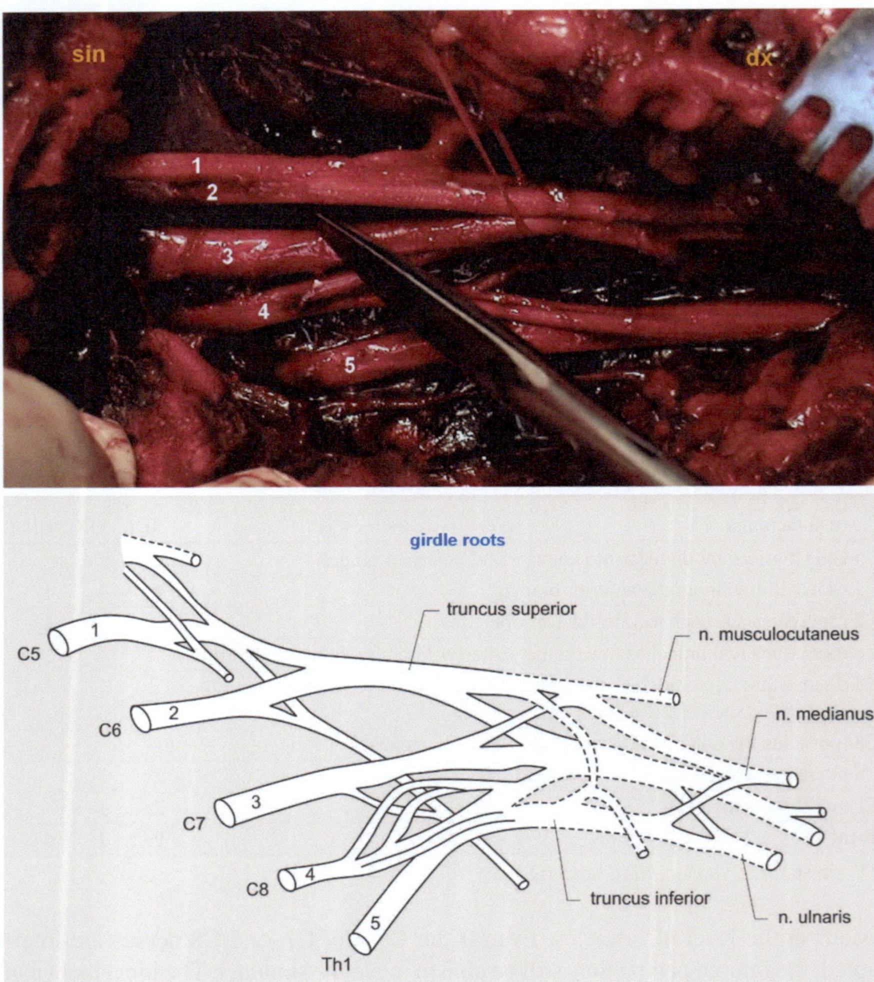

Fig. 4.4 Brachial plexus of the left side. From left to right, the C5 root (1), C6 root (2), C7 root (3), and C8 root (4) are divided into more branches, T1 root (5) is thicker than the C8 root (photo captured by Prof. Viktor Matejčík, scheme illustrated by Mrs. Anna Francová)

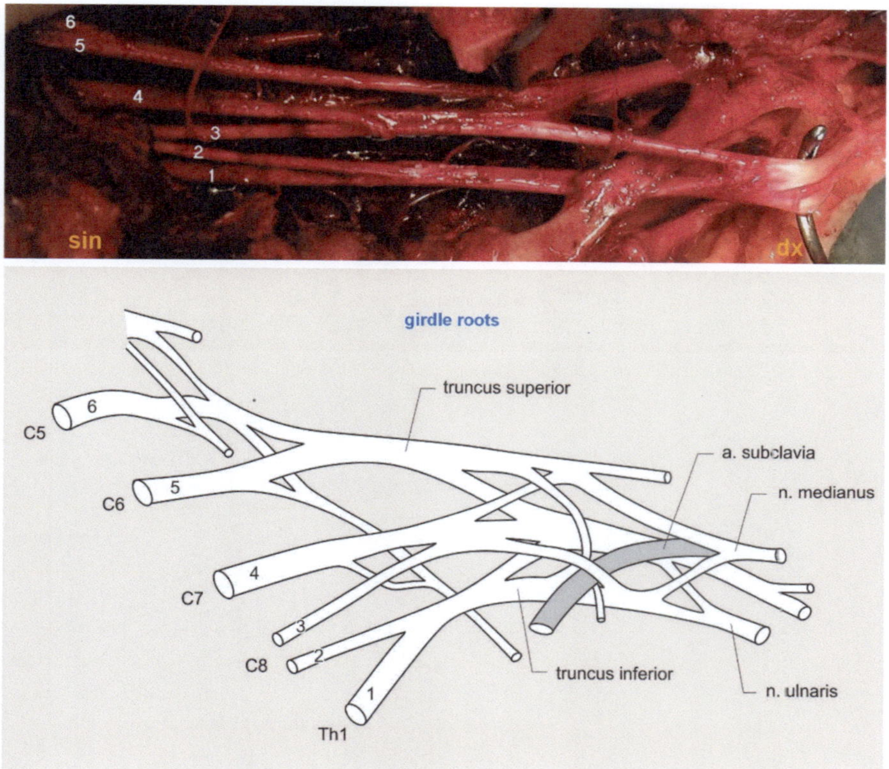

Fig. 4.5 Brachial plexus, left side. From left to right, the T1 root (1), and C8 root split into two branches (2, 3), C7 root (4), C6 root (5), C5 root (6), the branch of C8 root (2) joins T1 root (1); the branch of C8 root (3) connects to T1 root above subclavian artery (a. subclavia) (photo captured by Prof. Viktor Matejčík, scheme illustrated by Mrs. Anna Francová)

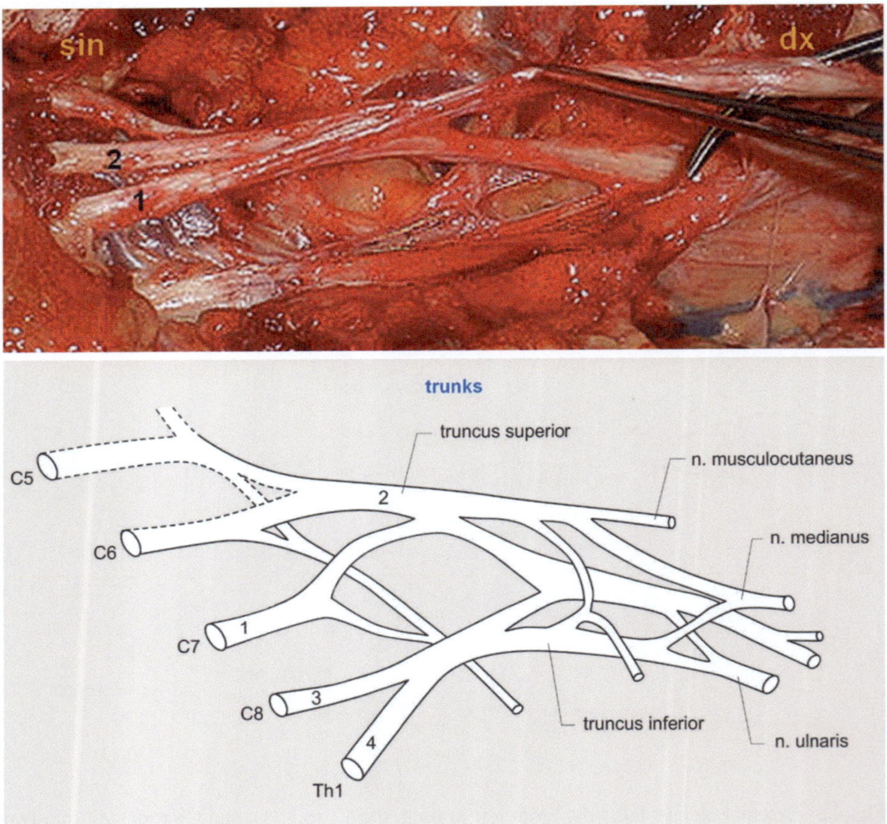

Fig. 4.6 Brachial plexus, left side. From left to right, the convergence of the C7 root (1) to the superior trunk (truncus superior) (2), C8 root (3), and T1 root (4) (photo captured by Prof. Viktor Matejčík, scheme illustrated by Mrs. Anna Francová)

References

1. Tubbs RS, El-Zammar D, Loukas M, Cömert A, Cohen-Gadol AA. Intradural cervical root adjacent interconnections in the normal, prefixed, and postfixed brachial plexus. J Neurosurg Spine. 2009;11(4):413–6.
2. Pernkopf E. Atlas of topographical and applied human anatomy. In: Thorax and extremities, vol. 2. 2nd ed. Philadelphia, PA: W.B. Saunders Company; 1989. p. 1–308.

Chapter 5
Variations and Lesions of the Brachial Plexus at the Level of Nerve Trunks

Damage of the Superior Trunk (Truncus Superior) (C5–C6) Is Characterized by a Plegia—Lesion

1. The deltoid muscle (m. deltoideus)—innervated by branches from the axillary nerve (n. axillaris).
2. The brachioradialis muscle (m. brachioradialis)—innervated by branches from the radial nerve (n. radialis).
3. The biceps brachii muscle (m. biceps brachii)—innervated by branches from the musculocutaneous nerve (n. musculocutaneous).
4. The brachialis muscle (m. brachialis)—innervated by branches from the musculocutaneous nerve (n. musculocutaneous).
5. The supinator muscle (m. supinator)—innervated by branches from the radial nerve (n. radialis).

Lesion of the upper roots is characterized by combined damage of the axillary (n. axillaris) and musculocutaneous nerves (n. musculocutaneus) and partially radial nerve (n. radialis) (branches innervating the brachioradialis and supinator muscles). These muscles are connected to the fifth and sixth segments. The function of other muscles innervated by the radial nerve may not be affected.

In case of damage to the superior trunk, a lesion of the suprascapular nerve (n. suprascapularis) may be observed. Bicipital and tricipital reflexes are absent. With this lesion, the hand hangs next to the body, it cannot be rotated outwards, and the forearm cannot be flexed. The hand, wrist, and forearm are in pronation.

Superior trunk injuries can occur due to

1. Traction injuries during difficult birth with turning the head on the opposite side and pressing the shoulder on the same side.
2. Radiation injury.
3. Congenital lesion.

Z. Haviarová et al., *Peripheral Nervous System*,
https://doi.org/10.1007/978-3-031-73744-2_5

4. Tumours.

Adduction in the arm and its external rotation is impaired as a result of impaired innervation of the supraspinous muscle (m. supraspinatus) from the suprascapular nerve (n. suprascapularis) and infraspinous muscle (m. infraspinatus) from suprascapular nerve (n. suprascapularis). The loss of sensitivity spreads to the area of the deltoid muscle (m. deltoideus) and the radial part of the forearm.

Damage to the Middle Trunk (Truncus Medius) (C7) Is Characterized By a Lesion

1. Triceps brachii muscle (m. triceps)—innervated by the radial nerve (n. radialis).
2. The extensor carpi radialis muscle (m. extensor carpi radialis)—innervated by the radial nerve (n. radialis).
3. The extensor pollicis longus muscle (m. extensor pollicis longus)—innervated by the radial nerve (n. radialis).
4. The extensor digiti minimi muscle (m. extensor digiti minimi)—innervated by the radial nerve (n. radialis).
5. The extensor digiti communis muscle (m. extensor digiti communis)—innervated by the radial nerve (n. radialis).
6. The extensor carpi ulnaris muscle (m. extensor carpi ulnaris)—innervated by the radial nerve (n. radialis).
7. The flexor carpi radialis muscle (m. flexor carpi radialis)—innervated by the median nerve (n. medianus).
8. The flexor pollicis longus muscle (m. flexor pollicis longus)—innervated by the median nerve (n. medianus).
9. The pronator teres muscle (m. pronator teres)—innervated by the median nerve (n. medianus).
10. Opponens pollicis muscle (m. opponens pollicis)—innervated by the median nerve (n. medianus).

Damage of the middle trunk (truncus medius) is characterized by combined damage, especially the radial nerve (n. radialis) and partially median nerve (n. medianus) (outer lateral branch).

Incomplete damage to m. triceps, m. extensor, and m. abductor pollicis longus remains paralyzed, to which (in addition to fibres from the C7 root) nerve fibres from the C6 and C8 roots also arrive. Due to the damage of the median nerve (n. medianus), the pronation and opposition of the thumb are partially impaired, because their function is connected with the C7 segment. Reflex from the triceps brachii muscle is missing.

Damage of the Inferior Trunk (Truncus Inferior) (C8–T1) (Dejerine–Klumpke)

The lower trunk contributes to the three main nerves of the shoulder, and when damaged, each of them can show symptoms of disability [1]. Its contributions are complete to the forearm, and therefore, the muscles of the forearm and hand supplied by radial, ulnar, and median nerves (n. radialis, n. ulnaris, and n. medianus) can be affected.

The lesion of the inferior trunk (truncus inferior) consists of damage to the internal–medial branch of the median nerve (n. medianus), the entire ulnar nerve (n. ulnaris), and medial cutaneous brachial and antebrachial nerves (nn. cutanei brachii et antebrachii mediales).

It is characterized by damage and paralysis of muscles:

1. Extensor pollicis brevis muscle (m. extensor pollicis brevis)—innervated by the radial nerve (n. radialis).
2. The abductor pollicis muscle (m. abductor pollicis)—innervated by the radial nerve (n. radialis).
3. The flexor digitorum superficialis muscle (m. flexor digitorum superficialis)—innervated by the median nerve (n. medianus).
4. The pronator quadratus muscle (m. pronator quadratus)—innervated by the median nerve (n. medianus).
5. The palmaris longus muscle (m. palmaris longus)—innervated by the median nerve (n. medianus).
6. The radial half of the flexor digitorum profundus muscle (m. flexor digitorum profundus-pars radialis)—innervated by the median nerve (n. medianus).
7. The ulnar half flexor digitorum profundus muscle (m. flexor digitorum profundus-pars ulnaris)—innervated by the ulnar nerve (n. ulnaris).
8. The flexor carpi ulnaris muscle (m. flexor carpi ulnaris)—innervated by the ulnar nerve (n. ulnaris).
9. The adductor pollicis muscle (m. adductor pollicis)—innervated by the ulnar nerve (n. ulnaris).
10. Interossei muscles (mm. interossei)—innervated by the ulnar nerve (n. ulnaris).
11. Lumbrical muscles (mm. lumbricales)—innervated by the ulnar nerve (n. ulnaris).
12. Small muscles of the wrist—innervated by the ulnar nerve (n. ulnaris).

In the case of a lesion of the inferior trunk C8–T1, the function of the finger extensors innervated by the radial nerve is partially damaged. The function of basic muscles (innervated by the radial nerve) is preserved. The function of the muscles innervated by the median nerve (by its external–lateral branch) is preserved in this case. The function of the ulnar nerve and cutaneous nerves of the shoulder and forearm is completely damaged. The clinical symptomatology of this syndrome resembles the picture of mixed damage to the median and ulnar nerves. In this type of lesion, the function of the sympathetic fibres located mainly in the roots of C8 and

T1 is often disturbed. Lesions of the lower trunk often occur as a result of a traction lesion of the abducted upper limb during a difficult childbirth, tumours of the upper thoracic aperture, cervical rib, or radiation damage. In the clinical picture, there is a paresis of the flexion of the fingers and all muscles of the hand. Loss of sensitivity is on the ulnar side of the hand and forearm. Ipsilateral Horner's syndrome can occur with damage to the T1 root and the exit of preganglionic fibres from the superior cervical ganglion (ganglion cervicale superior), along with ptosis, miosis, and hemianhydrosis.

We noted several variants regarding the branches departing from the nerve trunks. More distal along the upper trunk is the space of the suprascapular nerve (n. suprascapularis); in three cases, it departed from the C5 root. Variations at the level of formation of nerve trunks were as follows: in three cases, the upper trunk was not formed; in one case, the C5 and C6 roots did not join; in two cases, the C5 and C6 roots were divided into anterior and posterior branches; and then, the anterior branches of C5, C6, and C7 and posterior branches of C5, C6, and C7 were joined. In two cases, the middle trunk converged and joined with the upper trunk. In three cases, it was connected to the lower trunk. In one case, it appeared as if all branches of the middle and lower trunk diverged from this junction, and the posterior fascicle was not formed. We observed the largest number of anatomical variations in the area of formation of the lower trunk. In one case, the lower trunk was not formed. The roots of C8 and T1 were parallel, and T1 was even thicker. Twice the middle trunk (C7) was divided not into two but into several branches. In one case, no posterior branch from the lower trunk was present (Table 5.1, Fig. 5.1).

Table 5.1 Variations of the brachial plexus at the level of plexus trunks and their branching

Type		SIN.	DX.	Bilat.
Superior trunk	C5 and C6 roots are divided into anterior and posterior divisions	2		
	C5 and C6 not connected	1		
	Formed by a small 2 mm junction of C5 and C6	1		
	C5 and C6 connected at the upper margin of the clavicle			1
Truncus medius	Connected to the superior trunk			2
	Connected to the inferior trunk	2	1	
	After issuing an anterior division toward the anterior division of the superior trunk, joining the posterior division of the superior and inferior trunk			1
Truncus inferior	C8 and T1 not connected	1		
	As a small 2 mm connection between C8 and T1	1		1
	Connected via two branches to the anterior and posterior division of the superior trunk	1		
	C8 joins T1 above the subclavian artery		1	
	Not issuing the posterior division		1	
	Formed only after 4 cm of the common course of C8 and T1	2	4	2
Total		**11**	**7**	**7**

SIN. sinister, *DX.* dexter, *Bilat.* bilateral

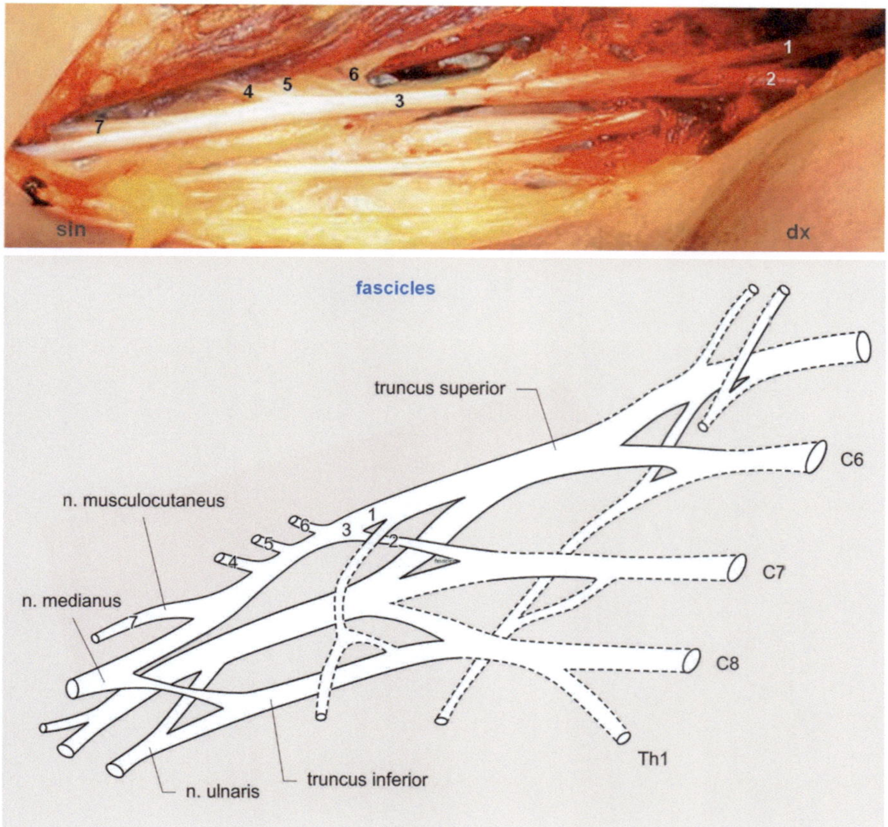

Fig. 5.1 Brachial plexus, right side. From right to left, the lateral root of the median nerve (1) is thicker than the medial one (2), the median nerve (3), branches to the biceps brachii muscle (4, 5, 6), and the musculocutaneous nerve (7) (photo captured by Prof. Viktor Matejčík, scheme illustrated by Ms. Anna Francová)

Reference

1. Shoja MM, Tubbs RS. Augusta Déjerine-Klumpke: the first female neuroanatomist. Clin Anat. 2007;20:585–7. https://doi.org/10.1002/ca.20474.

Chapter 6
Variations and Lesions of the Brachial Plexus at the Level of Nerve Fascicles

Damage to the posterior fascicle (fasciculus posterior) is characterized by a lesion of the axillary and radial nerves.

Damage to the medial fascicle (fasciculus medialis) is characterized by a lesion of the inner branch of the median nerve and to the ulnar nerve and medial cutaneous brachial nerve. The inner branch to form the median nerve receives fibres from C8 and T1 and provides innervation:

1. Flexor digitorum superficialis muscle.
2. Pronator quadratus muscle.
3. Palmaris longus muscle.
4. Flexor digitorum profundus muscle.

These muscles flex the wrist, the middle joints of II.–IV. finger, and the last phalanges of II.–III. finger.

Damage to the lateral fascicle (fasciculus lateralis) is characterized by a lesion of the musculocutaneus nerve and outer branches of the median nerve. The outer branch is supplied mainly from the C7 segment and provides innervation:

1. Flexor pollicis longus muscle.
2. Pronator teres muscle.
3. Opponens pollicis muscle.

The posterior fascicle (fasciculus posterior) supplies mainly flexors, and the medial and lateral fascicles supply the extensors.

The medial fascicle contributes to the innervation of the intrinsic muscles of the hand supplied by the median nerve, and the lateral fascicle contributes to the innervation of the sensory component of the median nerve. The presence of Horner's syndrome indicates the avulsion of the spinal roots C8, T1 [1].

Variations at the level of the plexus nerve fascicles were as follows: in four cases, the connection from the anterior branch of the superior trunk to the anterior branch of the middle trunk (truncus medius) was not formed. In one case, a lateral fascicle

Z. Haviarová et al., *Peripheral Nervous System*,
https://doi.org/10.1007/978-3-031-73744-2_6

was formed by a branch from the C8 root and in one case from the inferior trunk. In two cases, the lateral fascicle was formed by the anterior branch of the superior trunk. In cases where the middle truncus was divided into several branches, the additional ventral branch did not connect with the ventral branch of the superior trunk as usual but participated in the formation of the medial root of the fork of the median nerve. Variations of the lateral fascicle were common. We observed different combinations and mostly multiple connections between the lateral and medial fascicles, before the exits of the median and musculocutaneous nerves. Thanks to these connections, the medial root of the "fork" of the median nerve almost always contains fibres of the lateral fascicle, and in three cases also, the ulnar nerve receives fibres from the same fascicle at this level. The greatest variation in the formation of the nerve trunks was found in the lateral fascicle, which continues as the musculocutaneus nerve (C5, C6, C7) after the exit of the terminal branch of the median nerve.

The medial fascicle in cases where the C7 trunk is divided not into two—as usual—but into several branches receives fibres not only from C8, T1 (T2) but also from C7. It can also receive the same fibres from C7 in case of the presence of the lateral branch of the ulnar nerve. In two cases, a typical medial fascicle was not formed. The medial fascicle continued as the ulnar nerve after the exiting of the medial cutaneous antebrachial, the medial cutaneous brachial nerves (n. cutaneous antebrachii medialis, n. cutaneous brachii medialis), and the terminal branch of the medial root of the median nerve. The posterior branches of all three trunks formed the posterior fascicle. The posterior fascicle is usually the thickest of the plexus fascicles, formed by the union of sometimes not three but four branches. In most cases, the posterior branch of the upper trunk (C5, C6) is the thickest, and the posterior branch of the inferior trunk (C8, T1) is the thinnest in all cases. However, there were even more variations. In one case, the posterior branch of C7 was thin, and there was no connection with the posterior branch of the upper trunk, but only with the thin branch that diverged from it; the axillary nerve or the subscapular nerve (nervus subscapularis) and the thoracodorsal nerve (n. thoracodorsalis) were not present. These branches diverged from the posterior branch of the superior trunk, which continued as the axillary nerve to the quadrangular space (foramen quadrilaterum) (Table 6.1).

Table 6.1 Variations at the level of plexus fascicles

Type		SIN.	DX.	Bilat.
Lateral fascicle	Anterior divisions of C5, C6, and C7 connected in the lateral fascicle	1		
	Formed by the anterior division of the superior trunk		1	1
	Formed by the connection of the anterior divisions of the superior trunk and C8	1		
	Formed by the connection of the anterior divisions of the superior trunk and one division of the inferior trunk		1	
	Formed by the connection of the anterior divisions of the superior trunk and the anterior branch of C8 and C7		1	
	Issues branch to the medial branch of the median nerve	2	2	
	Formed by almost the whole anterior branch of C7 and issues a branch to the ulnar nerve	1	1	
Posterior fascicle	Posterior divisions of C5, C6, and C7 and the inferior trunk connected to form the posterior fascicle	1		
	Issues branches to the medial branch of the median nerve	1		
	Issues branches to the lateral branch of the median nerve	1		
	Misses the posterior division of the superior trunk	1		
	Formed low under the clavicle			1
	The posterior fascicle is formed by the whole posterior division of the superior trunk, which represents 90%, and one small thin division of the middle trunk		1	1
	Issues connections to the ulnar nerve			1
Medial fascicle	Receives the posterior division from the superior trunk	1		
	Formed by a separate branch of T1	1		
Total		**11**	**7**	**4**

SIN. sinister, *DX.* dexter, *Bilat.* bilateral

Reference

1. Traynelis VC, Malone HR, Smith ZA, et al. Rare complications of cervical spine surgery: Horner's syndrome. Glob Spine J. 2017;7(1_suppl):103S–8S. https://doi.org/10.1177/2192568216688184.

Chapter 7
Variations and Lesions at the Level of the Terminal Branches of the Brachial Plexus

Anastomotic branches from all three fascicles participate in the formation of the median nerve and more rarely the ulnar nerve (Tables 7.1 and 7.2).

Terminal Branches of the Brachial Plexus

Axillary nerve—C5–C6 arises from the posterior fascicle and provides abduction of the upper limb above the horizontal. Problems with abduction to the side and lifting of the arm forward and backward are associated with its lesion. It is flabby trying to lift the arm, and the entire shoulder rises. Later on, an atrophy of the deltoid muscle develops (Fig. 7.1).

Radial nerve—C5–T1 arises from the posterior fascicle, and the clinical picture depends on the level of the injury. In the case of an injury in the upper third of the shoulder, a picture of its complete deficit arises—plegia. There is an inability to extend the forearm, hand, and fingers in the metacarpophalangeal joints. In the case of a lesion of r. profundus, due to the shortening of the flexors, extension in the middle and distal joints of the fingers and abduction and adduction of the fingers innervated by the median and ulnar nerves are also impaired. The thumb is adducted to the index finger by the action of the functional adductor pollicis muscle (m. adductor pollicis) innervated by the ulnar nerve. In the case of a lesion of the radial nerve in the middle third of the shoulder, i.e., below the origin of the branch of the triceps brachii muscle, the function is preserved.

The C5–T1 radial nerve can be damaged in fractures of the middle part of the humerus, where the nerve is affected in the spirally running sulcus nervi radialis.

The terminal branches of the posterior fascicle were the most stable—for the radial nerve, in two cases, an anastomotic branch to the ulnar nerve was detected. In three cases, a deviation of the formation of the axillary nerve is a continuation of the

Z. Haviarová et al., *Peripheral Nervous System*,
https://doi.org/10.1007/978-3-031-73744-2_7

Table 7.1 Variations of the brachial plexus at the level of formation of terminal branches

Type		SIN.	DX.	Bilat.
Axillary nerve	Continuation of the posterior division of the trunk	3		
Musculocutaneous nerve	The lateral fascicle enters the coracobrachialis muscle, where the musculocutaneus nerve emerges and subsequently joins the median nerve in the lower third of the arm		1	
	Goes together with the median nerve, makes a fusion, and departs from the median nerve at various level	3	3	1
	Musculocutaneus nerve goes beside the biceps nerve and only issues branches	1		
	Issues anastomosis with the median nerve	3	2	1
Median nerve	Bifurcation of the median nerve is under the axillary artery		3	2
	The lateral part of the lateral fascicles is missing, the bifurcation is formed by a branch of C7	1		
	Formed by anastomotic branches from the lateral fascicle	2	1	
	Formed by anastomotic branches from the posterior fascicle	1	3	1
	Formed by anastomotic branches from the medial fascicle	6	3	1
	Formed in the lower half of the arm	6		3
Total		**27**	**16**	**9**

SIN. sinister, *DX.* dexter, *Bilat.* bilateral

Table 7.2 Variations of the brachial plexus at the level of formation of terminal branches

Type		SIN.	DX.	Bilat.
Radial nerve	Issues anastomosis to the ulnar nerve	1	1	
Ulnar nerve	A branch from the lateral fascicle participates in its formation	1	1	
	A branch from the posterior fascicle participates in its formation	1		
Cutaneous antebrachii medialis nerve	Anastomosis with the ulnar nerve	1		
Cutaneus brachii medialis nerve	Not formed	1	1	
Total		**5**	**3**	**0**

SIN. sinister, *DX.* dexter, *Bilat.* bilateral

posterior branch of the superior trunk. Thoracodorsal nerve had a different distance, either from the posterior fascicle or from the axillary nerve.

Damage to the nerve in the middle third of the forearm can cause the loss of finger extension. Branches to the wrist extensors originate in the upper part of the forearm. It is possible to proceed similarly for sensitivity disorders. The radial nerve ensures sensitive innervation of the dorsal side of the arm, forearm, and back of the

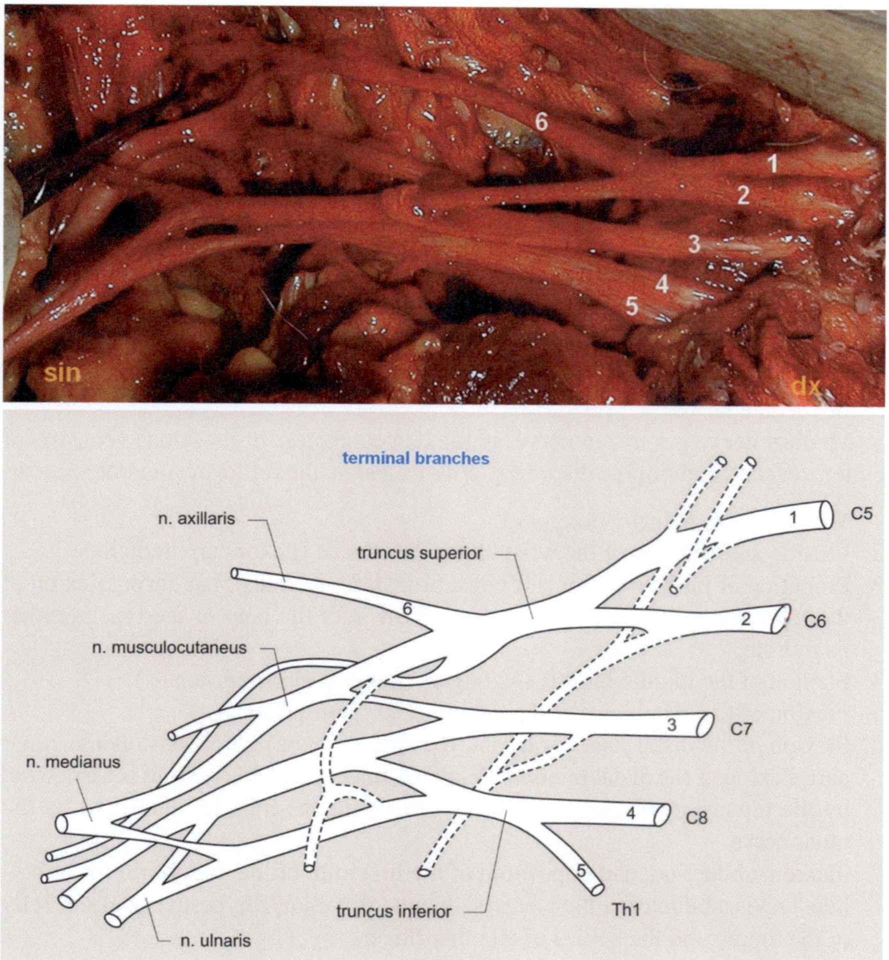

Fig. 7.1 Brachial plexus, right side. From right to left, C5 root (1), C6 root (2), C7 root (3), C8 root (4), T1 root (5), and axillary nerve (6)—continuation of the posterior branch of the superior trunk (photo captured by Prof. Viktor Matejčík, scheme illustrated by Mrs. Anna Francová)

hand, thumb, and II. and III. fingers, except for the last two phalanges of the middle and distal phalanx of the third finger. Its damage to the forearm results in a loss of sensitivity in the mentioned areas. Lesion of the radial nerve results in the following:

1. Paresis of flexion and extension of the elbow.
2. Supination of the forearm.
3. Extension of fingers and wrist.
4. Abduction of the thumb.

Musculocutaneus nerve—C5–C6 is a continuation of the lateral fascicle. It innervates the biceps brachii, coracobrachialis, and brachialis muscles. It flexes the shoulder and forearm and ensures supination of the forearm, elevation, and abduction of the shoulder. It can be damaged in humeral fractures, resulting in atrophy of the mentioned muscles, as well as weakness of flexion and supination of the shoulder. A loss of sensation on the lateral side of the forearm occurs.

The musculocutaneus nerve was missing in eight cases, and then, the lateral root of the "fork" of the median nerve was thicker. Generally, it was a fusion of both nerves creating the impression of a single trunk, which could be dissected and retrograde up to its distance from the top of the "fork" of the median nerve, forming a common trunk with it. The lateral root of the median nerve may originate from two or three branches and in some cases appears as a branch of the musculocutaneous nerve. In nine cases, a common trunk of the median nerve is formed in the lower half of the arm. In five cases, the axillary artery was located superficial to the "fork" of the median nerve.

Median nerve is a mixed nerve, so the clinical picture of its damage consists of motor, sensory, and trophic disorders. With its lesion, the following disorders occur:

1. Wrist flexion (palmaris longus).
2. Flexion and bending of the wrist on the radial side (flexor carpi radialis).
3. Pronation of the wrist (pronator teres, pronator quadratus), but during flexion of the forearm, indistinct pronation is possible with the help of the brachioradialis muscle.
4. Flexion of the middle joint II.–V. fingers (flexor digiti superficialis).
5. Flexion of the distal joint of the thumb (flexor pollicis longus).
6. Flexion of the distal joints of II. and III. finger (flexor pollicis profundus), ulnar part, flexion of the distal joints of IV. and V. fingers is preserved—it is carried out by the ulnar part of the flexor digitorum profundus muscle innervated by the ulnar nerve.
7. Flexion, abduction, and opposition of the first joint of the thumb (m. flexor pollicis brevis, abductor pollicis brevis, opponens pollicis), hypesthesia of the belly of the thumb and the bellies of all other fingers.

As a result of the antagonistic influence of the unaffected adductor pollicis muscle, the thumb is in close contact with the index finger and is in dorsal extension because of the action of the extensors. The absence of thumb opposition function reduces the patient to a phylogenetically lower level, resulting in an image of a "monkey hand". In monkeys, the thumb cannot be in the opposition necessary for grasping objects. This function is only possible in humans. In the case of a lesion of the median nerve in the middle and lower third of the forearm, paresis of the muscles of the thumb (opponens pollicis, abductor pollicis brevis, flexor pollicis brevis) is observed. The function of the other muscles is preserved because the nerve branches originate from them at the level of the medial epicondyle of the humerus and the upper third of the forearm.

A characteristic symptom of partial damage is causalgia and hypesthesia dolorosa in its territory. In these cases, movement disorders can be at the expense of pain—that is, defensive mobilization of the limb, not muscle weakness. Muscle-articular sensitivity is absent in the inter-articular joints of the index finger. In case of long-term damage to the median nerve, the muscles of the thumb atrophy, and the surface of the palm flattens. Hyperemia of the skin and sweating (especially in the area of the index and middle finger) are often observed. At other times, the skin is pale, anhidrosis and hyperkeratosis are present, and thin skin, cloudy nails, and sometimes wounds in the area of the last joint of the index finger are observed due to trophic disorders. The distal part of the median nerve is often damaged during compression because of swelling of the surrounding muscles, during repeated movements of the wrist, extension, or pressure, which are observed below the transverse carpal ligament (ligamentum carpi transversum). Lesions of the median nerve in this section can cause carpal tunnel syndrome, which consists of painful paresthesias or tingling in the innervation area of the median nerve (thumb, index finger, medial part of the middle finger), which can spread to the wrist to the flexor retinaculum (retinaculum flexorum). Persistent damage of the median nerve at this level affects motor axons and can lead to weakness of finger flexion, abduction, and opposition of the thumb. More proximal lesions of the median nerve cause weakness of forearm pronation.

Ulnar nerve—in two cases, we observed two roots in its formation, which started from the lateral and medial fascicles. They had the same dimensions and joined the ulnar nerve on the medial side of the axillary artery (art. axillaris). In one case, a branch from the posterior fascicle and a branch from the medial cutaneous antebrachial nerve (n. cutaneous antebrachii medialis) participated. In two cases, the anastomotic branch of the radial nerve also participated.

As a result of the lesion of the interosseus muscles (mm. interossei), there is hyperextension of the metacarpophalangeal joints and flexion of the distal joints, and the hand has a characteristic claw-like appearance due to the predominance of extensors. It is especially visible by IV. and V. fingers because the distal joints of the other fingers are largely innervated by the median nerve. With a nerve lesion in the middle and lower part of the forearm, the function of the flexor carpi ulnaris and flexor digitorum profundus muscles is not disturbed; that is why some movement of the fingers and wrist is possible in this case. Deep sensitivity is absent in the area of the little finger. Muscle atrophy of the adductor pollicis muscle (m. adductor pollicis), hypothenar muscles, and interosseous muscles are also present. Cyanosis, dryness, and cooling of the skin of the inner parts of the wrist, especially the little finger, are often observed. Trophic disorders include deformation of the little fingernail and loss of hair on the ulnar side of the dorsal surface of the hand. Damage to the ulnar nerve is evidenced by an incomplete range of motion, weakening of muscle strength compared to the healthy side, sensitivity disorders, and atrophy in typical areas. The ulnar nerve can be damaged by fractures, dislocation, subluxation, deformities, or compression in the cubital canal or ulnar canal at the wrist. The lesion leads to atrophy of the hand muscles and adduction and abduction of the fingers stagnate and results in a claw-like position of the fingers (caused by hyperextension of the fingers at the metacarpophalangeal joints). There is a loss of skin sensitivity on the dorsal and palmar surface of the medial side of the hand, on the little finger, and on the medial side of the ring finger (IV. finger).

Mutual Relation between the Median and Musculocutaneus Nerves in the Shoulder

In some cases (Fig. 7.2), the musculocutaneus nerve (1) as a separate nerve arising from the brachial plexus (plex. brachialis) is missing and is a branch of the median nerve. The "fork" is located low in such cases. The figure shows that two nerves of

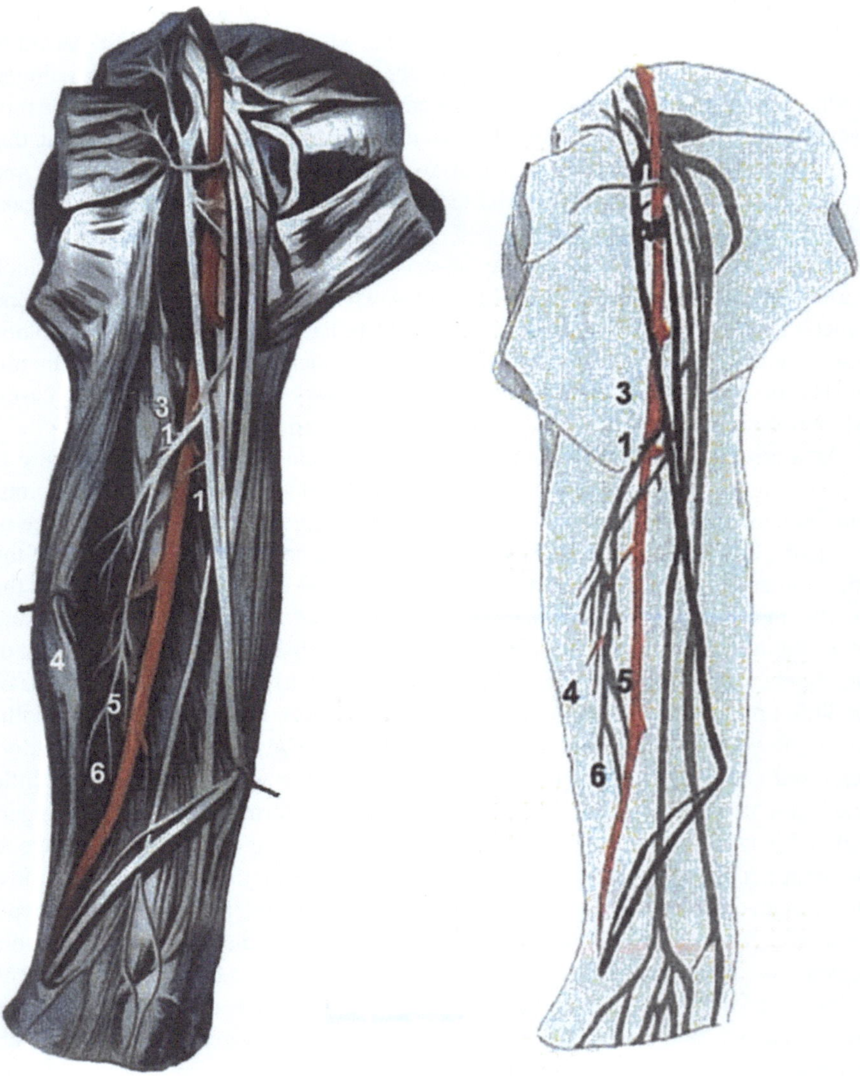

Fig. 7.2 Musculocutaneous nerve (1) as a separate nerve arising from the plexus brachialis is missing and is a branch of the median nerve, the "fork" is located low in such cases (illustrated by Mrs. Anna Francová)

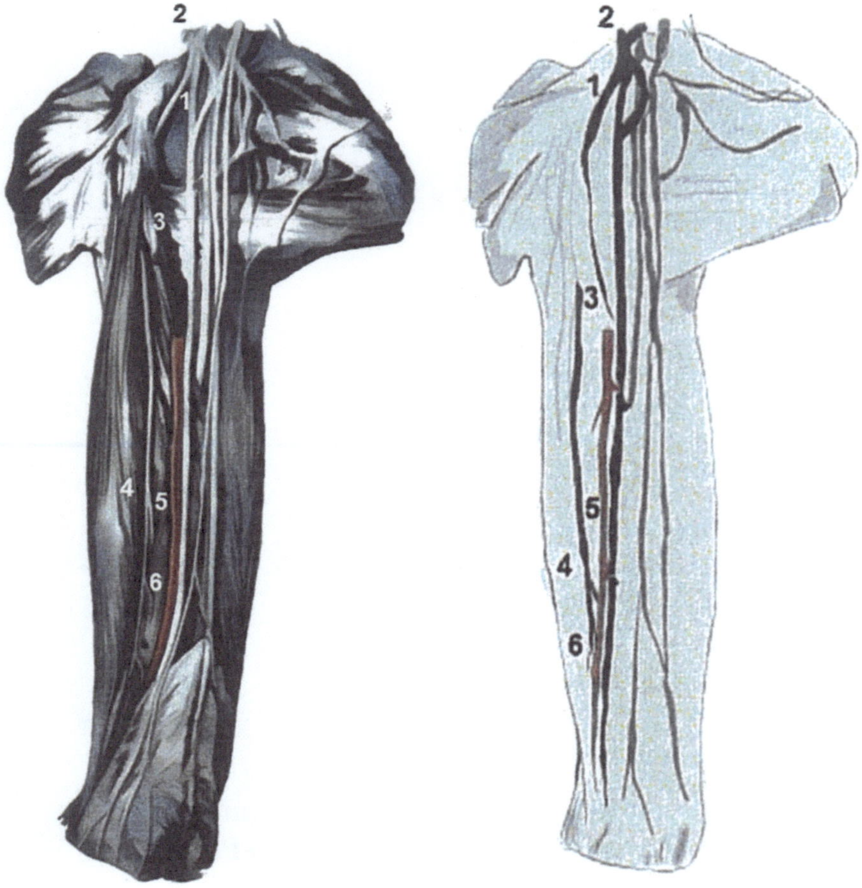

Fig. 7.3 When the "fork" is placed high, the median nerve comes out of the musculocutaneous nerve (1) separately from the plexus brachialis (illustrated by Mrs. Anna Francová)

different diameter exit from both "roots of the fork" above the coracobrachialis muscle (3) and merge into one trunk, from which the branches depart to the biceps brachii muscle (4) and to the brachialis muscle (5). The lateral cutaneous antebrachial nerve (n. cutaneous antebrachii lateralis) is a branch of the median nerve. In other cases (Fig. 7.3), in the high location of the "fork" of the median nerve, the musculocutaneus nerve (1) originates separately from the brachial plexus (2). It penetrates through the coracobrachialis muscle (3) and passes between the biceps brachii (4) and brachialis muscles (5), which it innervates. The final branch of this nerve is the lateral antebrachial cutaneous nerve (6). We also know another type of musculocutaneous nerve formation (Fig. 7.4).

The described anatomical differences point to the fact that with severe damage to the median nerve, there also are symptoms of damage to the musculocutaneous nerve present.

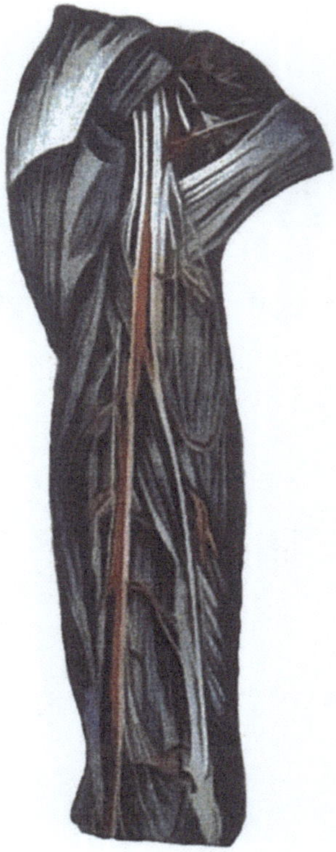

Fig. 7.4 Another type of arrangement (illustrated by Mrs. Anna Francová)

Differences in Construction of the Posterior Antebrachial Interosseus Nerve (N. Interosseus Antebrachii Posterior)

At the level of origin of the posterior antebrachial interosseus nerve (n. interosseus antebrachii posterior), which is a continuation of r. profundus of the radial nerve (8), the nature of its branching and the connections with neighbouring nerves are unstable. Figs. 7.5 and 7.6. show the extensor digitorum communis muscle (m. extensor digitorum communis) (1) removed almost entirely and the supinator muscle (m. supinator) (2) partially discised. The tendons of the extensor pollicis longus (m. extensor pollicis longus) (3), extensor indicis (m. extensor indicis) (4), and abductor pollicis longus muscles (m. abductor pollicis longus) (6) were left unchanged, and dorsal carpal ligament (ligamentum carpi dorsalis) was cut.

In some cases (Fig. 7.5), there is a considerably high level of origin (in the canalis supinatorius) of the posterior interosseus nerve (n. interosseus posterior) (8) from the deep branch of the radial nerve (9). Many neural branches are observed in the lower third of the forearm departing from it. Multiple conjunctions with r. superficialis of the radial nerve and r. profundus of the ulnar nerve were observed. The final branches of the posterior interosseus nerve (n. interosseus posterior) reach the carpal bones and carpometacarpal joints.

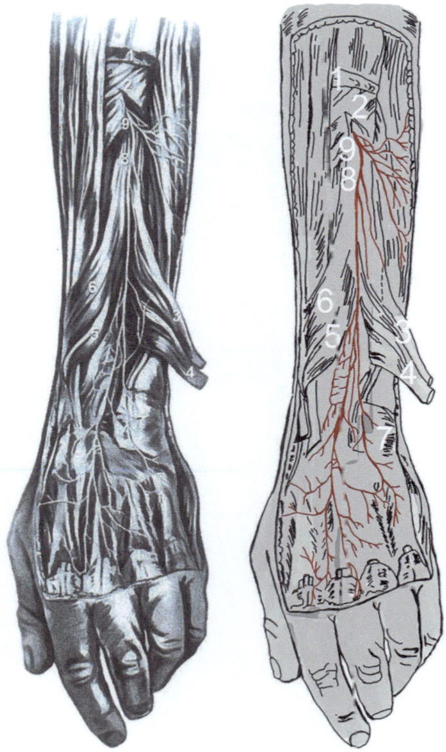

Fig. 7.5 High origin (in the canalis supinatorius) posterior interosseus antebrachial nerve (n. interosseus antebrachii posterior) (8) from the deep branch of the radial nerve (9), many nerve branches are observed in the lower third of the forearm, which depart from it (illustrated by Mrs. Anna Francová)

In other cases (Fig. 7.6), the posterior interosseus antebrachial nerve (n. interosseus antebrachia posterior) departs from the deep branch of the radial nerve in the lower section of the canalis supinatorius, while the final branches in the carpometacarpal junction are missing. Connections between the posterior interosseus nerve (n. interosseus antebrachia posterior) and neighbouring nerves are almost completely missing. Another type of formation of this nerve is in the next figure (Fig. 7.7).

Lesion of r. profundus of the radial nerve manifests itself by pain and weakness in the muscles innervated by it. It occurs in patients who perform a repeated movement-pronation-supination, which leads to repeated compression of the nerve by the fibrous edge—Frohse's ligament (proximal edge of the m. supinator). Extensor carpi radialis longus and brevis muscles (m. extensor carpi radialis longus et brevis) and brachioradialis m. are innervated by branches of the radial nerve departing before the formation of r. profundus of the radial nerve. In this case, no sensory deficit is present.

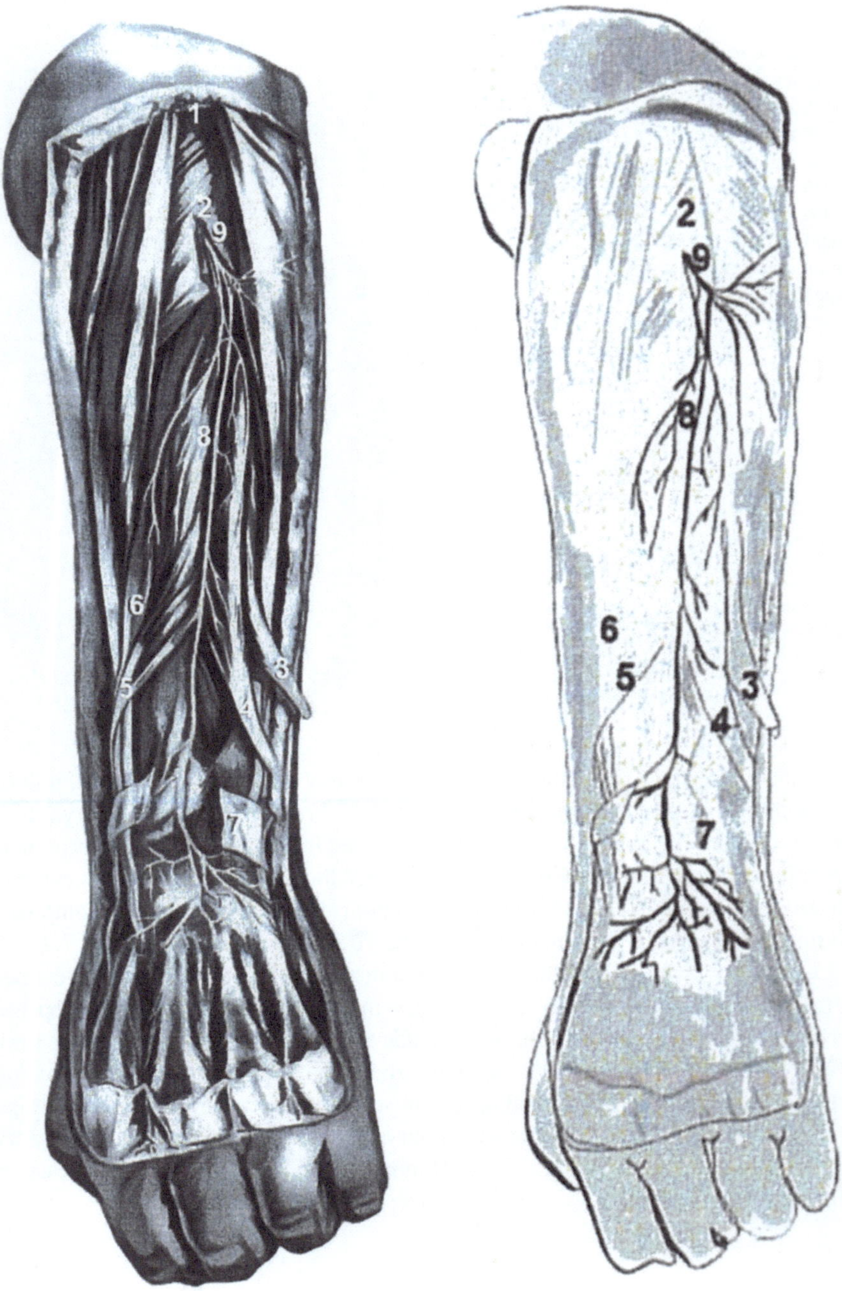

Fig. 7.6 The posterior interosseous antebrachial nerve departs from the deep branch of the radial nerve in the lower section of the canalis supinatorius; the final branches in the carpometacarpal junction are missing (illustrated by Mrs. Anna Francová)

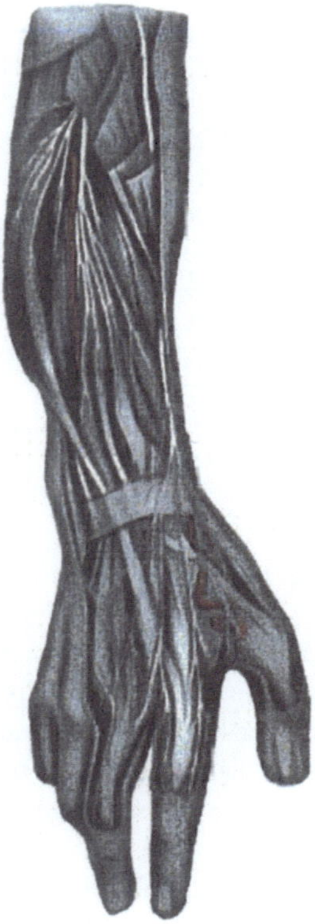

Fig. 7.7 Another type of formation (illustrated by Mrs. Anna Francová)

Brachial Plexopathies

The most common causes of brachial plexopathy are trauma, genetic mutations, primary autoimmune processes, radiotherapy, and neoplastic infiltration (Fig. 7.8). Diabetes mellitus is a potential factor in the development of lumbosacral plexopathies, less often in brachial plexopathies. Neoplastic plexopathies start with sharp pain and last days and weeks, which are followed by the development of muscular weakness with intervals of several weeks. Plexopathies are characterized by asymmetric weakness of the muscles of the limb and sensory deficits that do not correspond to the distribution of individual roots or nerves. Brachial plexopathies cause weakness of the shoulder girdle and arm muscles if the inferior and middle trunks of the plexus are involved. Sensory disturbances are variable but follow a simple pattern of the medial part of the plexus lesions e.g., tingling and numbness of the fourth and fifth fingers [3, 4]. Autonomic disorders caused by the interruption of sympathetic fibres from the brachial plexus passing through the lower trunk to the superior cervical ganglion may include trophic changes in the skin, oedema reflex sympathetic dystrophy (regional pain complex syndrome), and Horner's syndrome.

During movement of the head or shoulder, the brachial plexus must move freely within the surrounding tissues, like the peripheral nerves during movements of the

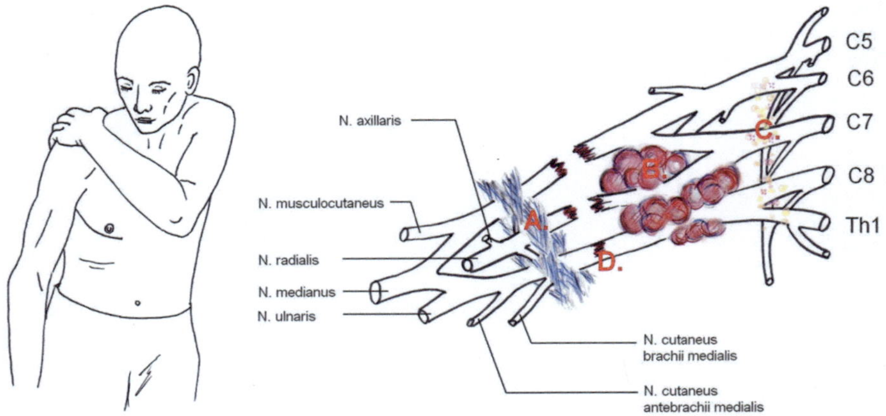

Fig. 7.8 Brachial plexopathy—clinical symptoms (illustrated by Mrs. Anna Francová)

limb. Freedom for this movement is provided by the loose connective tissue—the mesoneurium, which spreads between the epifascicular epineurium and connects the nerve trunk to the surrounding tissues, such as tendons, vessels, fascicular surfaces, and periosteum. In normal nerves, it is soft and sufficiently transparent, and it carries arteries and veins related to the vascular system of the nerve. It is usually thinned above and below each lesion site. Fibrotic changes of the mesoneurium, formed after an injury, are initiated by the formation of oedema or haematoma and are much more pronounced in the case of infection. They result in various parts of the plexus or peripheral nerves adhering to the surrounding tissue and being subjected to compression and traction for chronic scarring. They are more serious in areas where the ability to move is essential, especially in places specific to potential entrapment syndromes. Chronic compression can lead to changes in the small vessels of the endoneurium and perineuria with later perineural and endoneurial fibrosis. The more severe the injury, the more likely scar tissue will form in the nerve. To protect the fascicles against compression, the nerve trunk can shrink and change its shape. Individual fascicles of the nerve trunk can move freely one upon another to adapt to pressure and movement.

Peripheral nerves can be compressed at two levels of scarring: superficially by surrounding structures and intrafascicularly by fibrotic compression of axons. Early treatment of nerve damage, mostly performed by external neurolysis, is usually the initial step in most surgeries. It is recommended due to the development of posttraumatic fibrosis. It creates basic conditions for shortening the time required for the functional adjustment of the nerve after posttraumatic axonotmesis. After operations with a longer time interval, fibrotic tissue accumulates around the nerve, which sometimes has a cartilaginous consistency, which makes identification of the nerve difficult. In children, scar tissue formation is usually less pronounced and less compressive than in adults [1, 2] (see also Part VI, Chap. 18: Figs. 18.7–18.20).

References

1. Zvěřina E, Stejskal L. Poranění periférních nervů. Praha: Avicenum; 1979. p. 303.
2. Haninec P, Kaiser R. Operační léčba poranění plexus brachialis. ČSl Neurol Neurochir. 2011;74/107(5):619–30.
3. Swell RS. Clinical anatomy by regions. 7th ed. Baltimore: Livingstone; 2004. p. 991.
4. Kapeller K. Štruktúra autonómneho nervového vlákna. Bratislava: Veda; 1979. p. 160.

Chapter 8
Differences in the Structure of the Lumbosacral Plexus

The lumbosacral plexus is an analogue of the brachial plexus. Differences in the formation of the lumbosacral plexus, like the brachial plexus in the periphery, manifest themselves in such a way that the segmental participation of certain nerves, as well as the share of tissue innervation, can change.

We observed anatomical variations of the lumbosacral plexus in 50 cadavers. We monitored the extraforaminal deviations of the formation of individual roots on their terminal branches as well as the participation of the T12 and L4 or L5 roots in the formation of the plexus.

In all cadavers, the lumbosacral plexus was visualized bilaterally from the anterior approach. The lumbar plexus was visualized after the dissection of the psoas major muscle.

The lumbar plexus is formed in the psoas major muscle by the ventral branches of L1–L4 with or without T12 contribution [1–3]. The main bilateral lumbar nerve plexus and its branches were located along the surface of the most dorsolateral part of the vertebral body and intervertebral discs. The lumbar plexus is located laterally from the intervertebral foramina and passes through the psoas major muscle. The nerves of the sacral plexus are located on the frontal surface of the piriformis muscle (m. piriformis). The branches of the iliac vessels are near the roots of S1, S2, and S3. The sacral plexus is formed by the ventral branches of S1–S3 with the contribution of S4, and the important lumbosacral trunk (truncus lumbosacralis) is formed by the roots of L4 and L5. The border root involved in the formation of plexuses is the L4 root, which in some cases is largely involved in the formation of the lumbar plexus and other cases in the sacral plexus. The L4 root does not always play the role of the boundary root, and sometimes, it is the L5 root. As in the upper extremity, some trunks of the lower extremity receive more fascicles from higher nerves in the high cranial form than in the low caudal form. In the prefixed type, the T12 and L1 roots are thicker. Then, the L4 root contributes significantly to the sacral plexus, and the S3 and S4 roots are absent. The participation of the L4 root in the formation of the sacral plexus was in all our cases. In no case did we encounter a missing

Z. Haviarová et al., *Peripheral Nervous System*,
https://doi.org/10.1007/978-3-031-73744-2_8

connection between the plexuses. The prefixed type occurred in two cases and postfixed in one case. In the case of the prefixed plexus, a thick lumbosacral trunk was present, and only the S1 and S2 roots were present when the sacral plexus was formed, and the sacral plexus nerves diverged from the L5, S1, and S2 roots.

In the postfixed type, the lumbosacral trunk was thin, and the roots S3, S4, and S5 were also present (Fig. 8.1a, b). In the postfixed type, the S3 root may have the number of fibres normally carried in the S2 root, and the S4 contribution may be greater [1–5]. We never observed the occurrence of a prefixed plexus on one side and a postfixed one on the other. Root lesions differ from damage to individual nerves—then, the plegia is usually partial and depends on the segmental innervation of the muscles. While the S3 root commonly innervates the flexors of the thumb and rarely other limb muscles, the S4 root does not innervate any muscles in the limb. The coccygeus plexus (S5–Co) serves as a purely somatosensitive innervation of the skin around the coccyx. Sometimes, there is a connection from S4 and sometimes from S3. This small braid is placed on the coccygeus muscle (m. coccygeus), and motor fibres emerge from it. This contributes to the innervation of levator ani (m. levator ani) and coccygeus muscles and the anococcygeal nerves (nn. anococcygei) (Table 8.1).

Differences in the Structure of the Lumbar Plexus (Plexus Lumbalis)

In some cases (Fig. 8.2), the branch from T12 to L1 participates in the formation of the lumbar plexus, in addition to the branches still present connecting segments L1–L4. Then, the following nerves arise from it: accessory ilioinguinal nerve (n. illioinguinalis accessorius) (5), accessory femoral nerve (n. femoralis accessorius) (9), accessory obturator nerve (n. obturatorius accessorius), etc. In such cases, in the subinguinal area as well as in other areas, there are multiple connections between the nerves arising from the lumbar plexus. Figure 8.2 shows connections (9) between the lateral cutaneous femoral nerve branch, the iliohypogastric nerve (r. cutaneous femoris lateralis, n. iliohypogastricus), and the ilioinguinal nerves, between them and lateral cutaneous femoral nerve (n. cutaneous femoris lateralis) (16). In these cases, the branch from L4, which participates in the formation of the lumbosacral plexus, is thin (14).

Added explanations to Fig. 8.2. are as follows: 1—the intercostal nerve (n. intercostalis) XII, 2—iliohypogastric nerve, 3—lateral cutaneous branch (r. cutaneous lateralis) of the iliohypogastric nerve, 4—the ilioinguinal nerve, 6—the lateral cutaneous femoral nerve (n. cutaneous femoris lateralis), 7—anterior cutaneous branch (r. cutaneous femoris anterior) of the femoral nerve, 8—the femoral nerve (n. femoralis), 10—the obturator nerve, 11—the genitofemoral nerve (n. genitofemoralis), 12—the ilioinguinal nerve, and 13—external spermatic nerve (n. spermaticus externus).

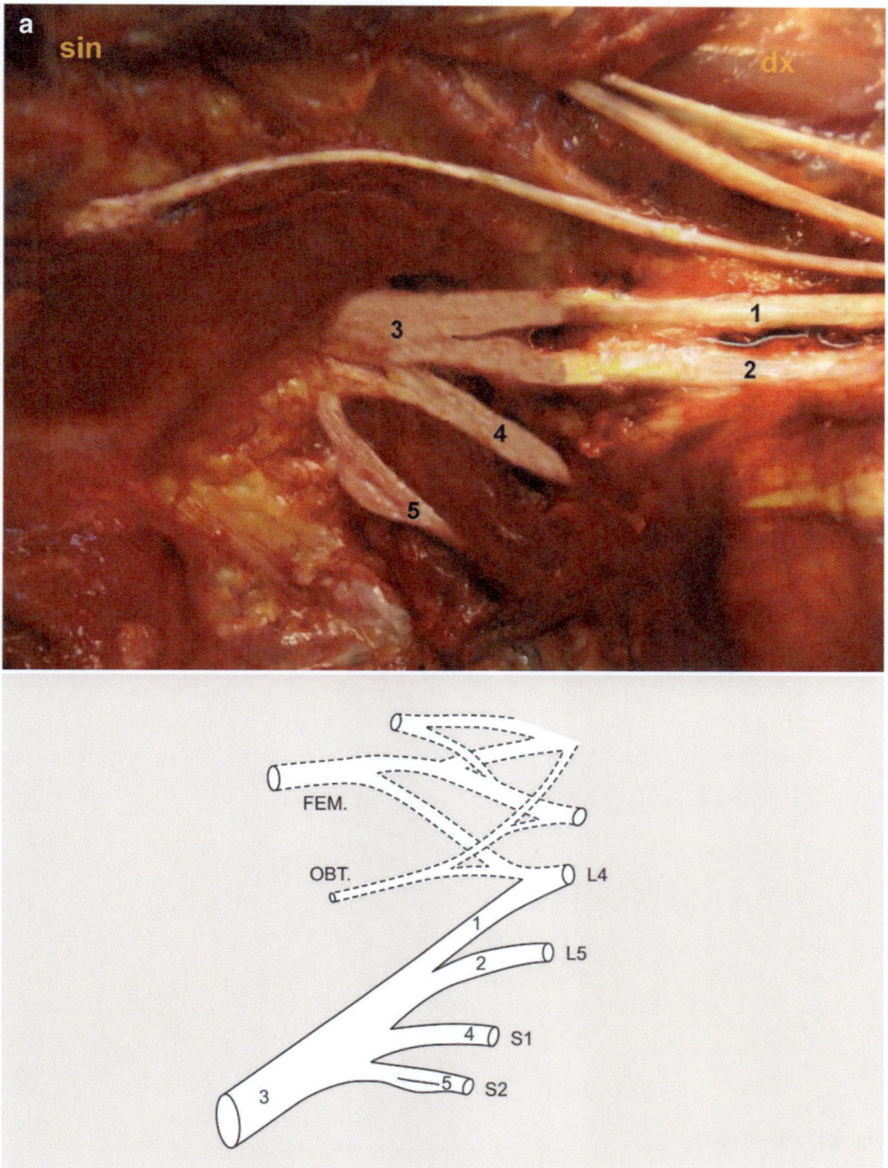

Fig. 8.1 (**a**) Prefixed type of lumbosacral plexus (plexus lumbosacralis), right side. Anterior view, the craniocaudal direction (right to left)—the branch from the L4 root (1) is thicker than the L5 root (2), thick lumbosacral trunk (truncus lumbosacralis) (3), S1 root (4), S2 root (5) (photo captured by Prof. Viktor Matejčík, scheme illustrated by Ms. Anna Francová). (**b**) Postfixed type of lumbosacral trunk (plexus lumbosacralis), front view, right side, craniocaudal direction (right to left). In the formation of the pudendal nerve (n. pudendus), the S3 root is mainly involved. A thin branch from the L4 root (1) to the L5 root (2), lumbosacral trunk (3), S1 root (4), S2 root (5), S3 root (6), S4 root (7), pudendal nerve (8), obturator nerve (9), femoral nerve (10) (photo captured by Prof. Viktor Matejčík, scheme illustrated by Ms. Anna Francová)

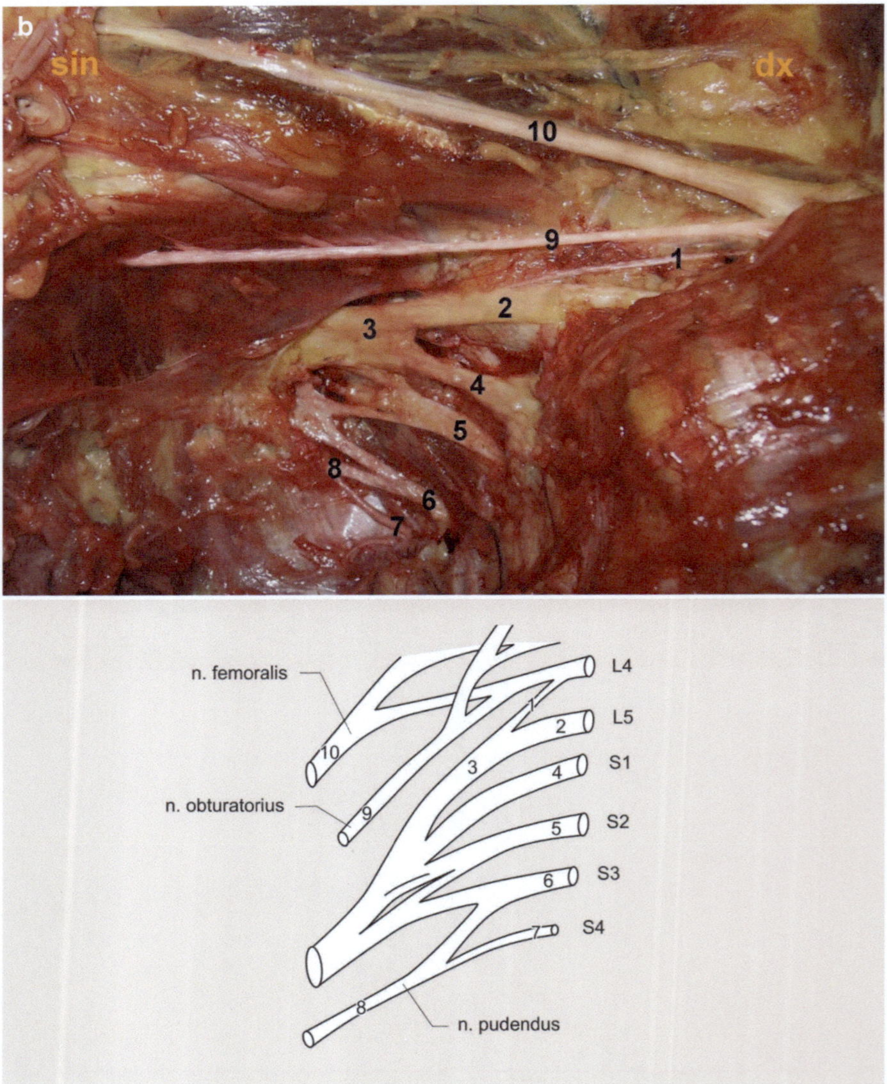

Fig. 8.1 (continued)

In other cases (Fig. 8.3), the connections from T12 to L1 are missing. Not only additional nerve trunks are missing, but also some important trunks/nerves (e.g., n. cutaneous femoris lateralis). In such cases, the latter is a branch of the obturator nerve (n. obturatorius) (4).

Added explanations to Fig. 8.3 are as follows: 1—the intercostal nerve XII, 2—the iliohypogastric nerve, 3—the ilioinguinal nerve, 5—the obturator nerve, and 6—the external spermatic nerve.

Table 8.1 Variations of the lumbosacral roots

The LS root number	Duplicate root origin	Plexiform root origin
L2	2	–
L3	4	–
L4	25	5
Simultaneous L3 + L4	–	2
Simultaneous L3 + L4 + L5	2	–
L5	8	4
S1	16	–
S2	8	–
Simultaneous S1 + S2	4	–
S3	1	–
S4	–	–
Total	**70**	**11**

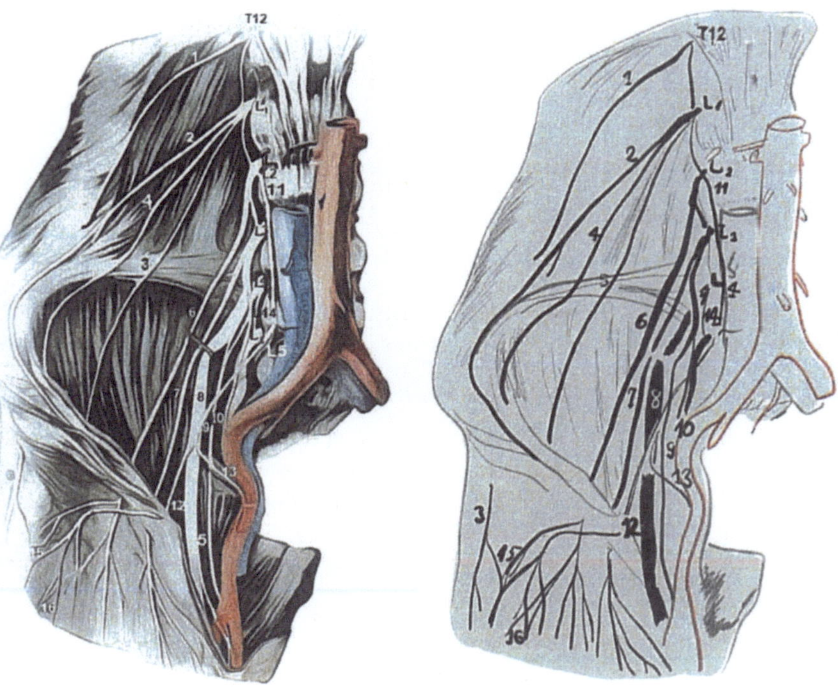

Fig. 8.2 The branch from T12 to L1 takes part in the formation of the lumbar plexus (illustrated by Mrs. Anna Francová)

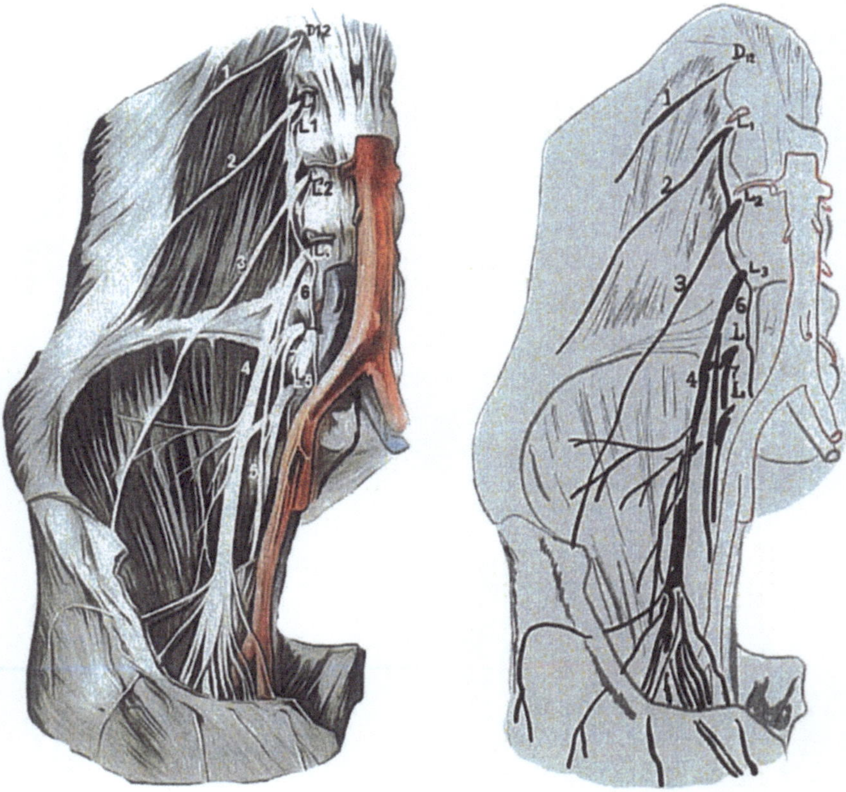

Fig. 8.3 The connection from T12 to L1 is missing on the plexus lumbar formation (illustrated by Mrs. Anna Francová)

Anastomoses between nerve trunks in the periphery are rare. The connecting branch participating in the formation of the lumbosacral trunk is generally well developed (7) (in Fig. 8.4.—another type of formation of the lumbar plexus) (see also Part VI, Chap. 18, Fig. 18.21, 18.22 and 18.23).

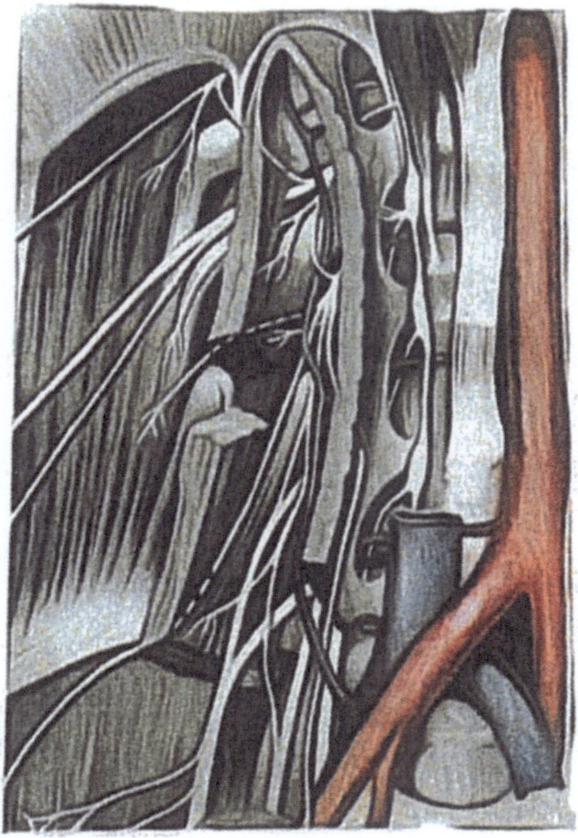

Fig. 8.4 Another type of the lumbar plexus formation (illustrated by Ms. Anna Francová)

Differences in the Structure of the Sacral Plexus (Plexus Sacralis)

There are multiple connections in the formation of the sacral plexus (L4–S3) (Fig. 8.5). With the formation of peripheral nerves, the posterior cutaneous femoral nerve (n. cutaneous femoris post.) (5), pudendal nerves (n. pudendus) (6), superior gluteal nerve (n. gluteus sup.) (1), inferior gluteal nerve (n. gluteus inf.) (2), and the branches of the plexus are involved, which in the proximal section are connected by multiple anastomoses. At the same time, a high division of the sciatic nerve (n. ischiadicus) into the common peroneal (n. peroneus communis) (3) and the tibial nerves (n. tibialis) (4) is observed. At other times, the presence of a double posterior cutaneous femoral nerve (n. cutaneous femoris posterior) is observed (5).

In other cases (Fig. 8.6), a different picture is observed. The branches from which the sacral plexus is formed run in isolation, and there are few connections between them. Likewise, a small number of connections are observed between the branches from which peripheral nerves are formed: the superior gluteal nerve (1), inferior

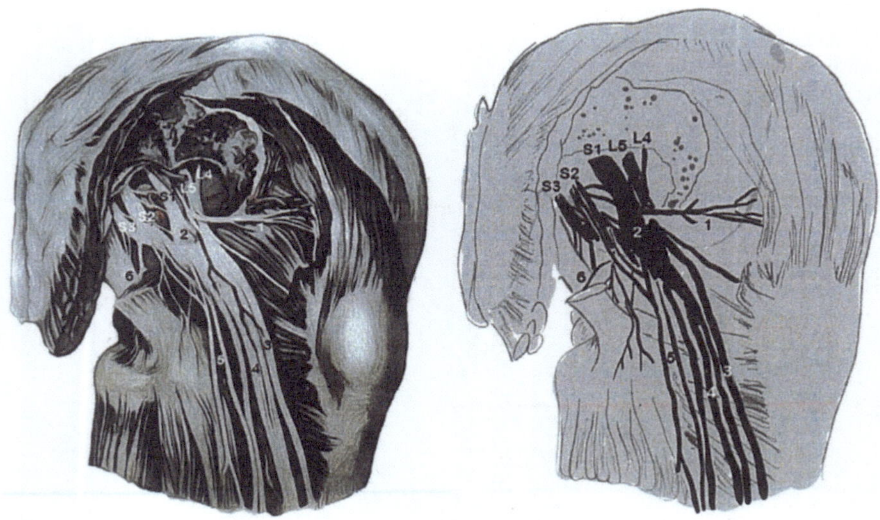

Fig. 8.5 In the formation of the sacral plexus (plexus sacralis) (L4–S3), there are multiple connections, at the same time a high division of the sciatic nerve (n. ischiadicus) to the common peroneal nerve (n. peroneus communis) (3) and tibial nerve (n. tibialis) (4) (illustrated by Mrs. Anna Francová)

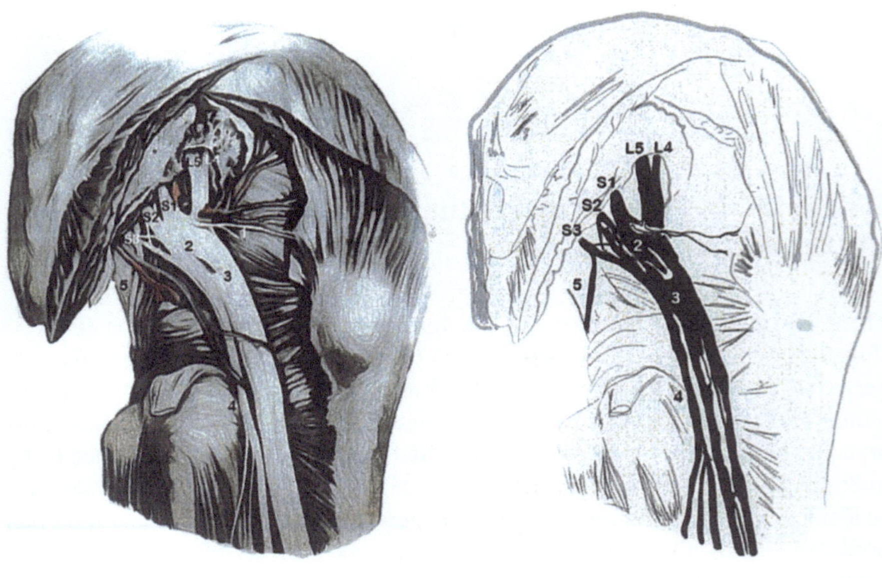

Fig. 8.6 The branches of the sacral plexus are isolated, and there are few connections between them. In such cases, the sciatic nerve usually divides low (illustrated by Mrs. Anna Francová)

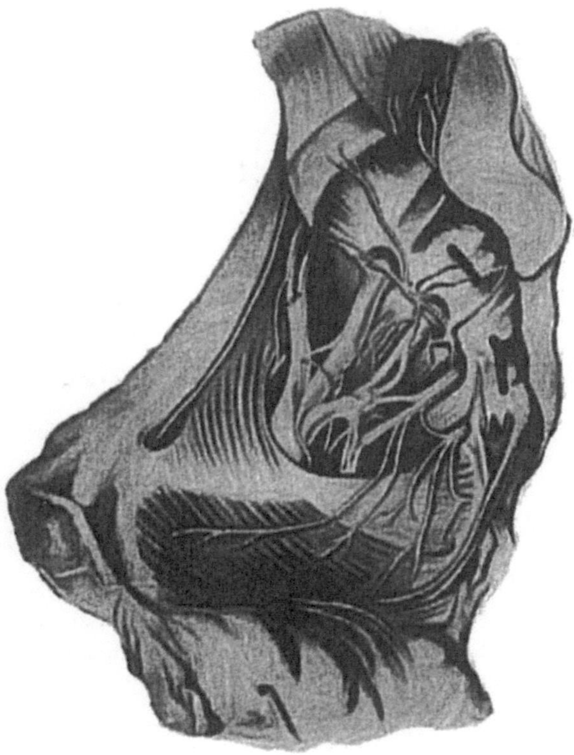

Fig. 8.7 Another type of sacral plexus formation (illustrated by Ms. Anna Francová)

gluteal nerve (2), posterior cutaneous femoral nerve (4), and pudendal nerve (5). The sciatic nerve (n. ischiadicus) (3) is usually divided low in such cases. After the removal of the epineurium, one can observe intersegmental junctions in the borders of the roots and plexuses, as well as in the periphery. We also observed another type of sacral plexus formation (Fig. 8.7).

Differences in Formation of the Obturator Nerve (N. Obturatorius)

In the formation of the obturator nerves (Fig. 8.8), the branches from the roots L1 and L5 can also participate. In some cases, the participation of the upper branches of the lumbosacral plexus prevails (Fig. 8.8), there is a high division of the basic trunk into terminal branches, and the presence of the accessory obturator nerve (n. obturatorius accessories) (6) (Fig. 8.8) is observed. Another type of obturator nerve forming is illustrated in the following picture (Fig. 8.8).

In other cases, branches from the lower lumbar roots take part in the obturator nerve formation (Fig. 8.9). In these cases, the low division into final branches is

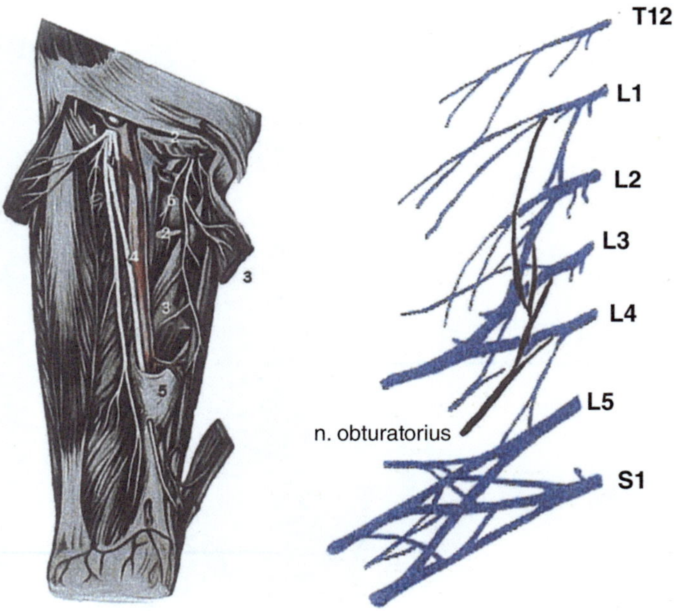

Fig. 8.8 In the formation of the obturator nerve (n. obturatorius), the participation of the upper branches of the lumbosacral plexus prevails. There is a high division of the basic trunk into terminal branches, and the presence of accessory obturator nerves (nn. obturatorii accessorii) is often observed (6) (illustrated by Ms. Anna Francová)

observed (Fig. 8.9). In some cases, branches from the roots L1, L2, L3, and L4 take part in its formation; in other cases, the branches from the roots L2, L3, L4, and L5 take part (Fig. 8.8) (see also Part VI, Chap. 18: Figs. 18.21, 18.22 and 18.23).

Added explanations to Figs. 8.8 and 8.9 are as follows: 2—pectineus muscle (m. pectineus), 3—adductor longus muscle (m. adductor longus), 4—the saphenous nerve (n. saphenous), and 5—vastoadductor membrane (lamina vastoadductoria) (Fig. 8.10).

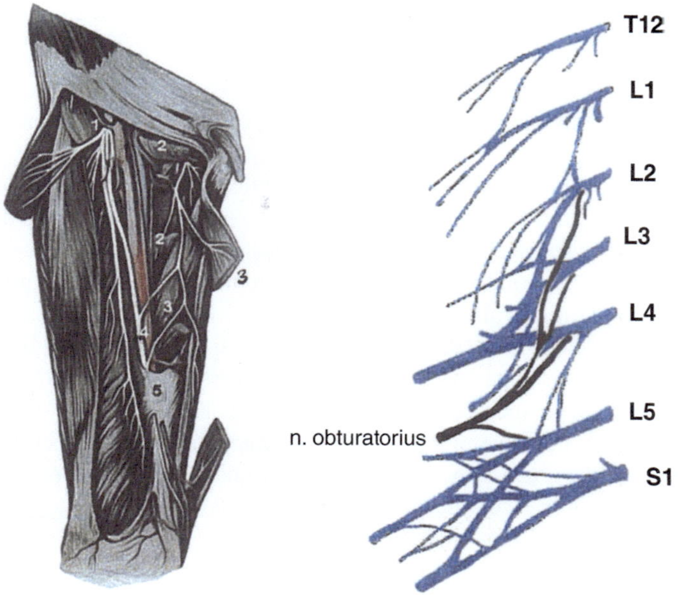

Fig. 8.9 In the formation of the obturator nerve (n. obturatorius), mainly branches from the lower lumbar roots are involved. In such cases, its low division into final branches is observed (illustrated by Ms. Anna Francová)

Fig. 8.10 Another type of formation of the obturator nerve (illustrated by Ms. Anna Francová)

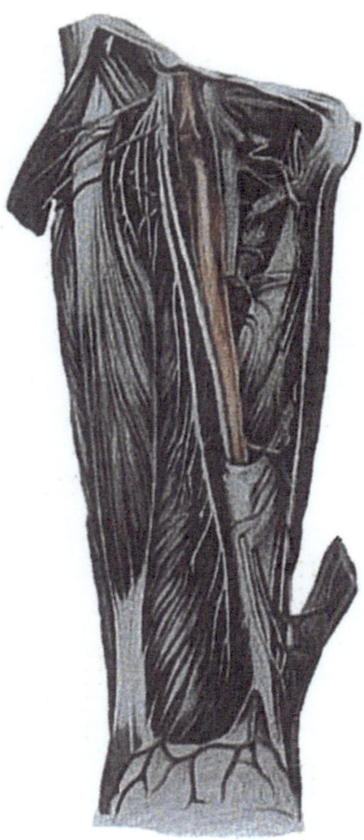

Differences in Formation of the Sciatic Nerve (N. Ischiadicus)

Figure 8.11 shows a high division of the sciatic nerve (n. ischiadicus), tibial nerve (n. tibialis, portio tibialis) (2), and common peroneal nerve (n. peroneus, portio peronealis) (3).

In such cases, the formation of the abovementioned nerves occurs in the sacral plexus (Fig. 8.11), and even on the thigh, they are separate trunks, between which anastomoses are almost absent. In such a construction/formation of the sciatic nerve, muscle branches originate high, and after removing the epineurium, they can be dissected up to the sacral plexus.

In other cases (Fig. 8.12), the sciatic nerve emerges from the pelvis as a single trunk, and only in the upper part of the popliteal fossa (fossa poplitea), it divides into final branches. In such cases, the sacral plexus seems to pass into one trunk (Fig. 8.12), within the range of which there are many internal connections. Muscle branches arise at the place of their exit from the trunk of the sciatic nerve, and therefore, it is not possible to dissect them from it. We also observed another type of formation (Fig. 8.13) of the sciatic nerve.

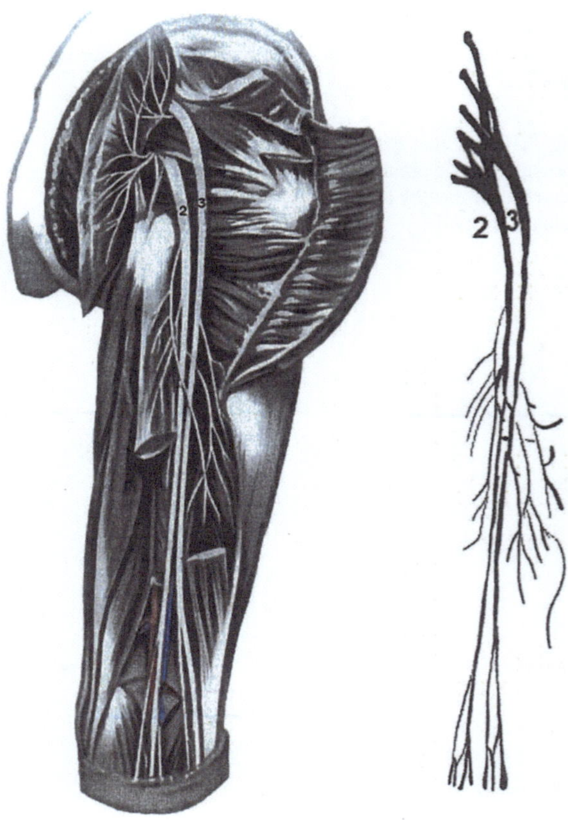

Fig. 8.11 High division of the sciatic nerve into the tibial nerve (2) and common peroneal nerve (n. peroneus communis) (3). The high division occurs in the sacral plexus. The muscle branches depart high (illustrated by Mrs. Anna Francová)

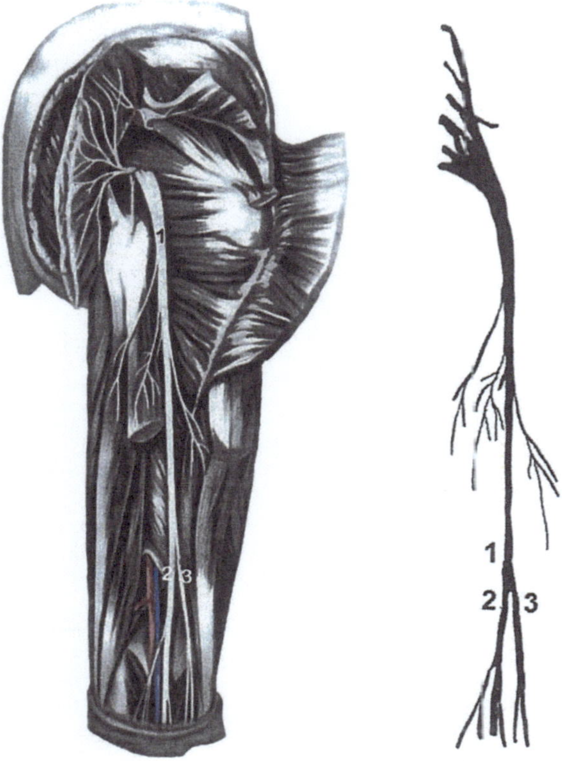

Fig. 8.12 The sciatic nerve emerges from the pelvis as one trunk, and only in the upper part of the popliteal fossa (fossa poplitea), it divides into final branches. Muscle branches arise at the place of their exit from the trunk of the sciatic nerve, and therefore, it is not possible to dissect them from it (illustrated by Ms. Anna Francová)

The low division may be caused by the presence of the epineurium, common to both parts of the nerve, and after removing it, we can divide both trunks to the place of their origin. In such cases, from the outside, one nerve consists of two separate trunks, between which connections are practically absent. These anatomical differences in the structure of the sciatic nerve explain the instability of clinical symptoms when the nerve is damaged. Thus, with a high division, the damage to the trunk in the middle part of the thigh can be limited by the disruption of the integrity of one of its parts, which means that we can observe symptoms characteristic of the interruption of the tibial or common peroneal nerves (n. peroneus communis). With a low division, partial damage to the sciatic nerve at this level in the clinical picture may manifest mixed symptomatology.

During the internal preparation inside the sciatic nerve, we can observe its net-like structure. In some cases, after the removal of the epineurium, the sciatic nerve easily divides into the tibial and common peroneal nerves of the sacral plexus.

A relatively small number of anastomoses are observed inside the nerve trunk and muscle branches in cases of high division of the sciatic nerve form practically at the plexus itself and only rarely do they have anastomoses with basic trunks.

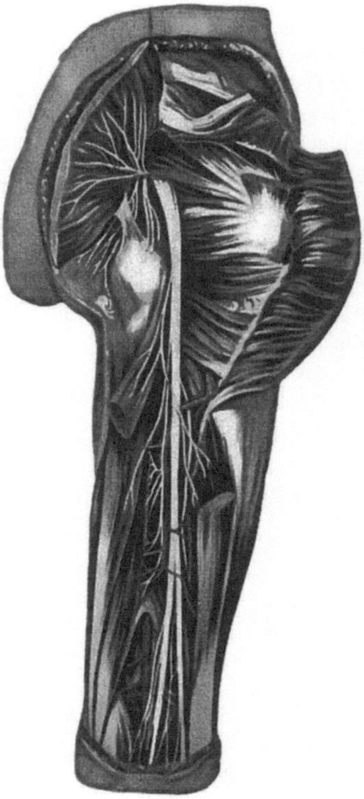

Fig. 8.13 Another type of formation of the sciatic nerve (illustrated by Ms. Anna Francová)

In other cases, after removing the epineurium, we can divide the sciatic nerve and observe many "anastomoses" between the tibial and deep peroneal (n. peroneus profundus) nerves.

The general nature of the structure of the nerve resembles a plexus, from which its components are formed in the upper part of the popliteal fossa, the muscle branches emerging from the trunk throughout its course. As a result, it is not possible to dissect these branches over a long distance without damage to the perineurium.

These differences in the structure of the nerve trunk reflect the diversity of the clinical picture that we observe in different people with sciatic nerve lesions at the same level. The obtained data point out the complexity and instability of the course of axons in the spinal nerves.

Variations in the region of the plexuses were frequently at the level of formation of nerve roots (Tables 8.1, 8.2 and 8.3). In 12 cases, we observed connections of the L3 root to the L4-L5-S1 roots.

In the lumbar plexus (Table 8.2), we observed a doubled exit of the roots in 33 and a plexiform exit in seven cases. In two cases, we observed an exit of three roots L2, L3, and L5 at the same time. Plexiform exit of the L4 root occurred in five cases and simultaneous exit of the L3 and L4 roots in two cases. We also observed changes in the sacral plexus (Table 8.3) at the level of the nerve roots in 41 cases. The double

Table 8.2 Variations of the lumbar roots

The L root number	Duplicate root origin	Plexiform root origin
L2	2	–
L3	4	–
L4	25	5
Simultaneous L3 + L4	–	2
Simultaneous L3 + L4 + L5	2	–
Total	**33**	**7**

Table 8.3 Variations of the sacral roots

The S root number	Duplicate root origin	Plexiform root origin
L5	8	4
S1	16	–
S2	8	–
Simultaneous S1 + S2	4	–
S3	1	–
S4	–	–
Total	**37**	**4**

exit of the L5 root in eight cases and the plexiform exit of the L5 root in four cases were observed. Double root exit of S1 after exit from the sacral foramina (foramina sacralia) in 16 cases, S2 in eight cases, and S3 in one case occurred. We observed the simultaneous exit of S1 and S2 roots in four cases. In 15 cases, the S1, S2, and S3 roots were divided at different distances after exiting from the sacral foramina. In two cases, the sciatic nerve was divided into tibial and peroneal portions already in the lower pelvis. The pudendal nerve was formed depending on the type of plexus from the S2 and S3 roots. Underappreciation of the importance of anatomical variability could be the cause of the failure of surgical treatment. Formation of the pudendal nerve depends on the type of plexus. When prefixed, the roots S1 and S2 were dominant in the formation of the pudendal nerve, and in postfixed, especially, the root S3 and to a lesser extent also S4 prevailed. The S2 root is mostly involved in the formation of the pudendal nerve, which is an important motor and sensory nerve to the pelvic organs and perineum. It also innervates the anal and urethral sphincters. Symptoms of the pudendal nerve lesion can also be caused by the S1 nerve root lesions. The different degree of damage depends on the representation of the individual roots S1–S4, according to the type of plexus and variations in the distance of the nerves (see also Part VI, Chap. 18: Figs. 18.21, 18.22, 18.23, 18.24, 18.25, 18.26, 18.27, 18.28, 18.29, 18.30, 18.31, 18.32, 18.33, 18.34, 18.35, 18.36, 18.37, 18.38, 18.39, 18.40, 18.41, 18.42, 18.43, 18.44, 18.45, 18.46 and 18.47) (Fig. 8.14, 8.15, 8.16, 8.17, 8.18, 8.19, 8.20 and 8.21).

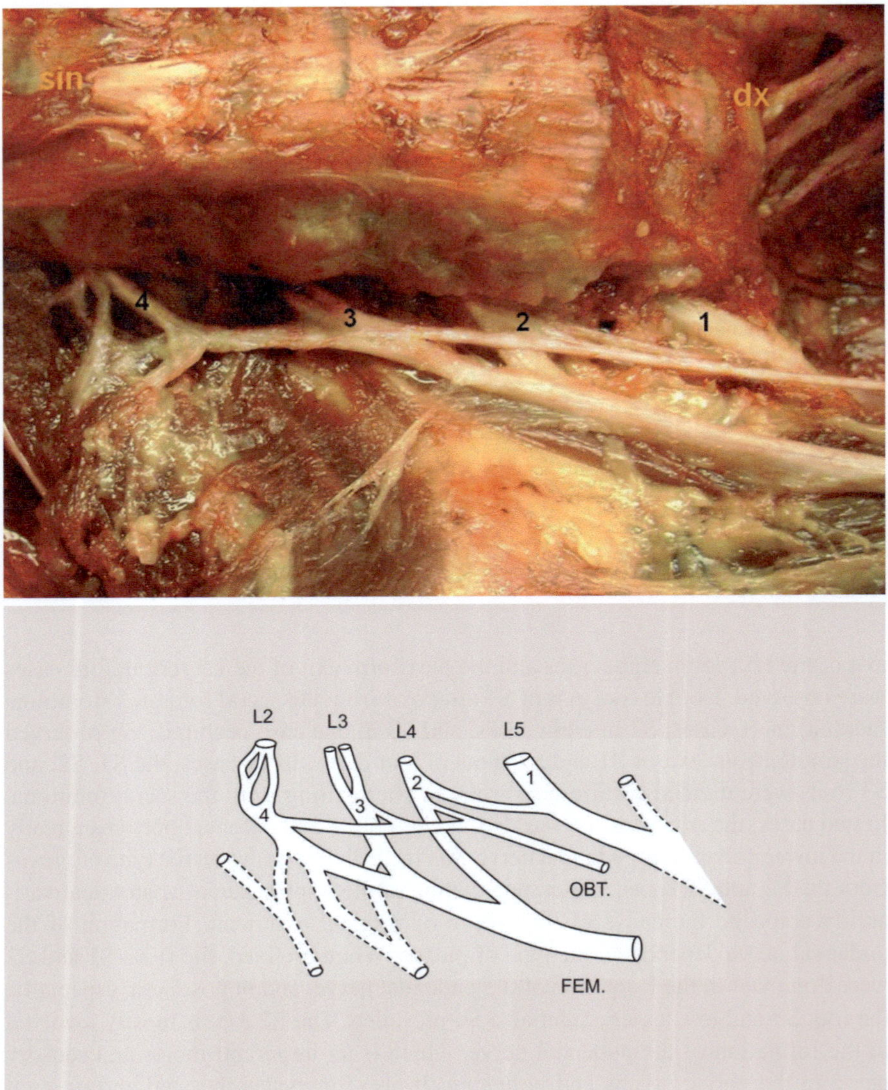

Fig. 8.14 Diverging exit of roots L2 and L3, right side. Front view, craniocaudal direction (left to right)—L5 root (1), L4 root (2), L3 root (3), L2 root (4) (photo captured by Prof. Viktor Matejčík, scheme illustrated by Ms. Anna Francová)

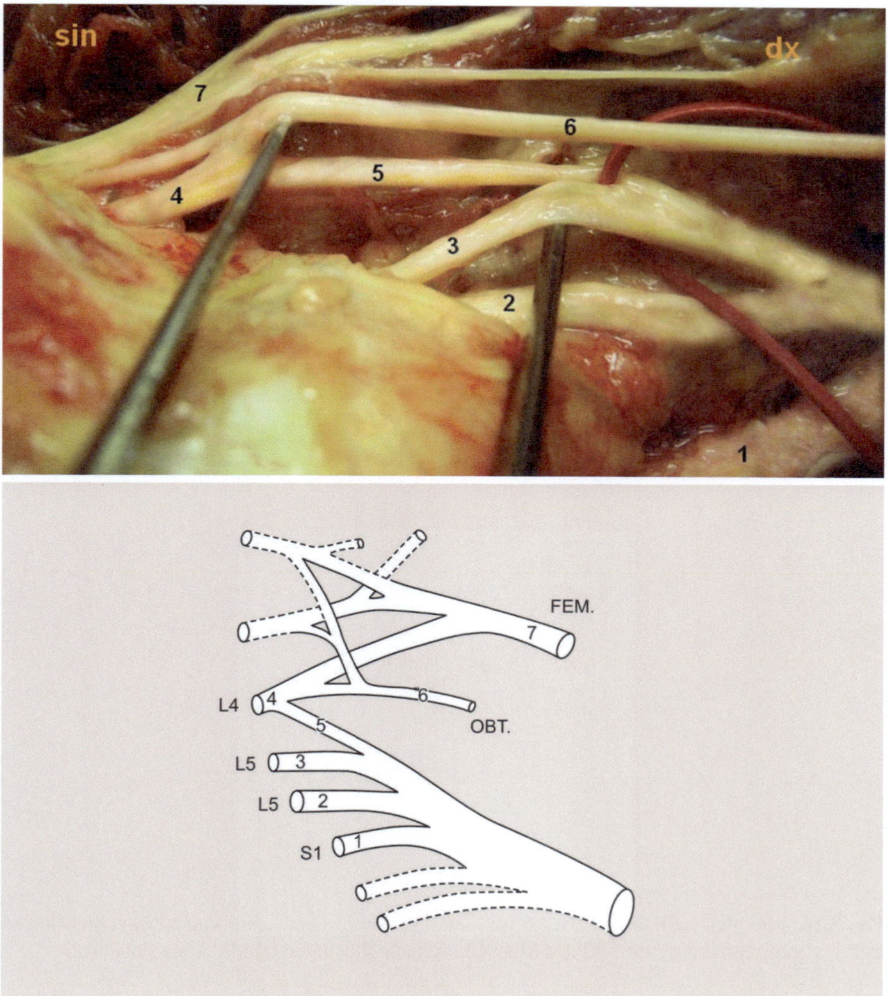

Fig. 8.15 The double exit of L5 root, left side. Front view, craniocaudal direction (from left to right)—S1 root (1), L5 root (5), obturator nerve (6), femoral nerve (7) (photo captured by Prof. Viktor Matejčík, scheme illustrated by Ms. Anna Francová)

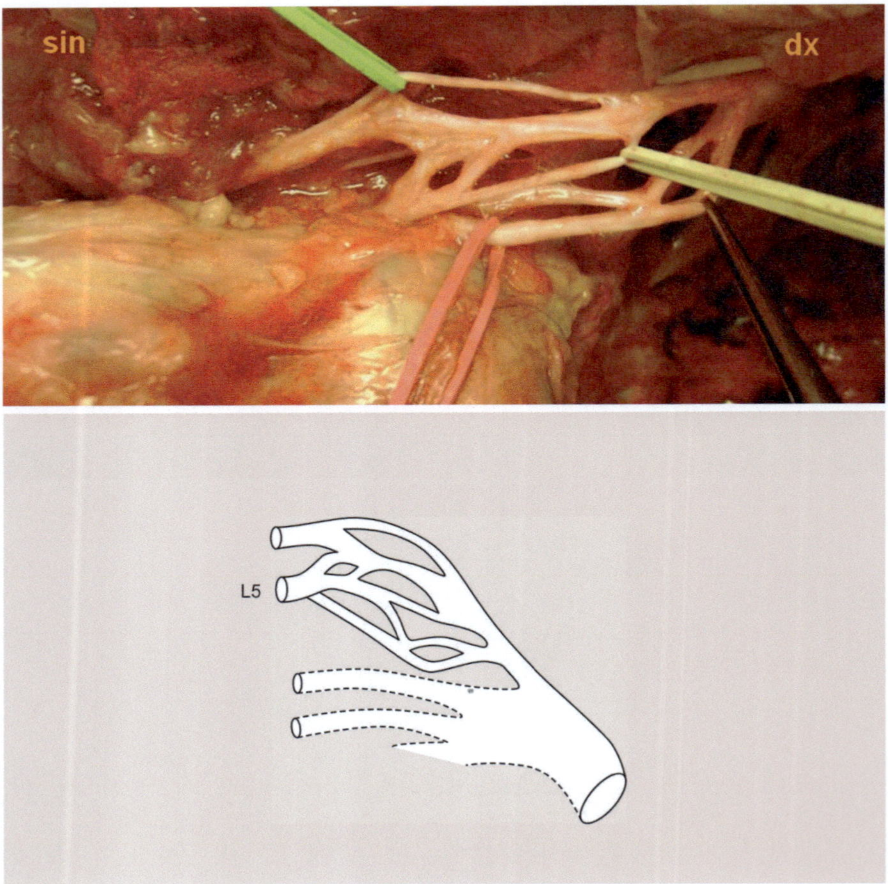

Fig. 8.16 The plexiform exit of the L5 root left side. Front view, craniocaudal direction (left to right) (photo captured by Prof. Viktor Matejčík, scheme illustrated by Ms. Anna Francová)

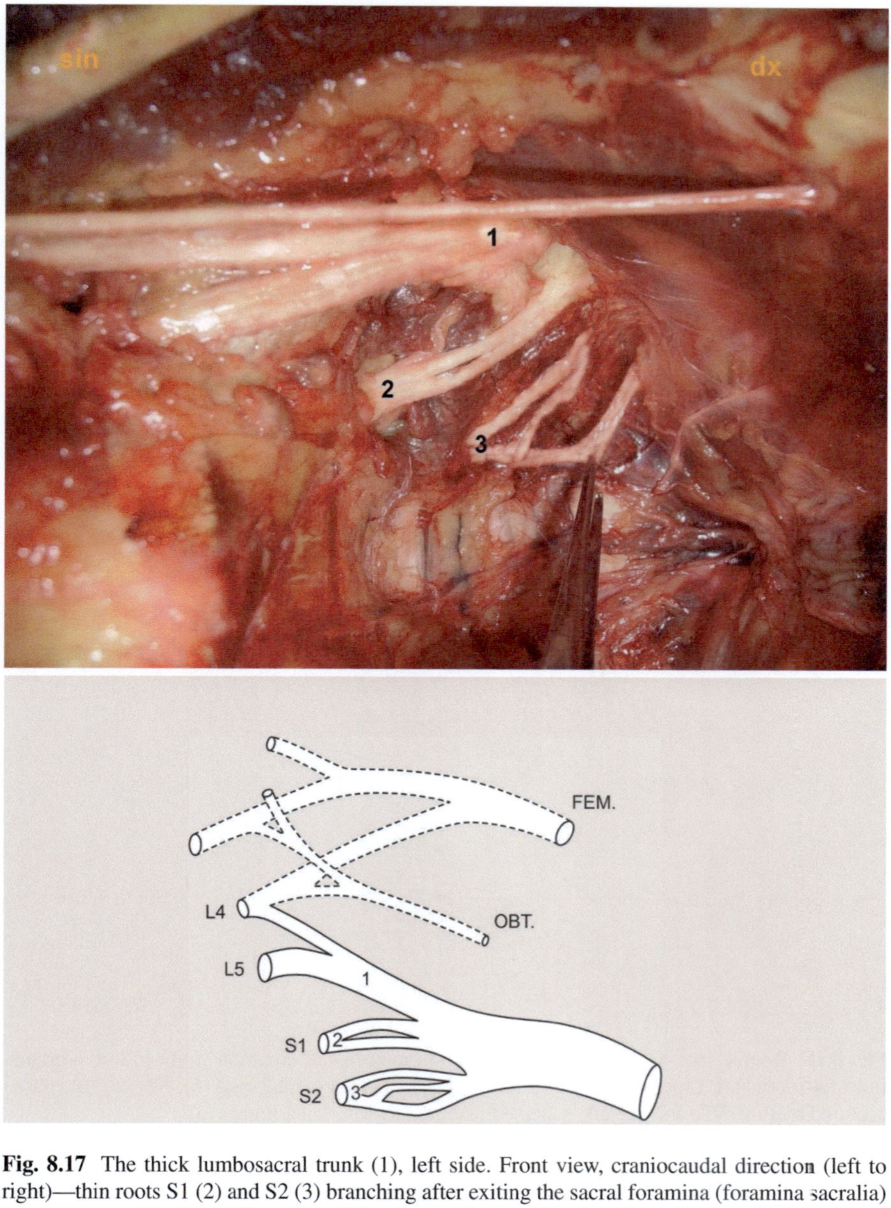

Fig. 8.17 The thick lumbosacral trunk (1), left side. Front view, craniocaudal direction (left to right)—thin roots S1 (2) and S2 (3) branching after exiting the sacral foramina (foramina sacralia) (photo captured by Prof. Viktor Matejčík, scheme illustrated by Ms. Anna Francová)

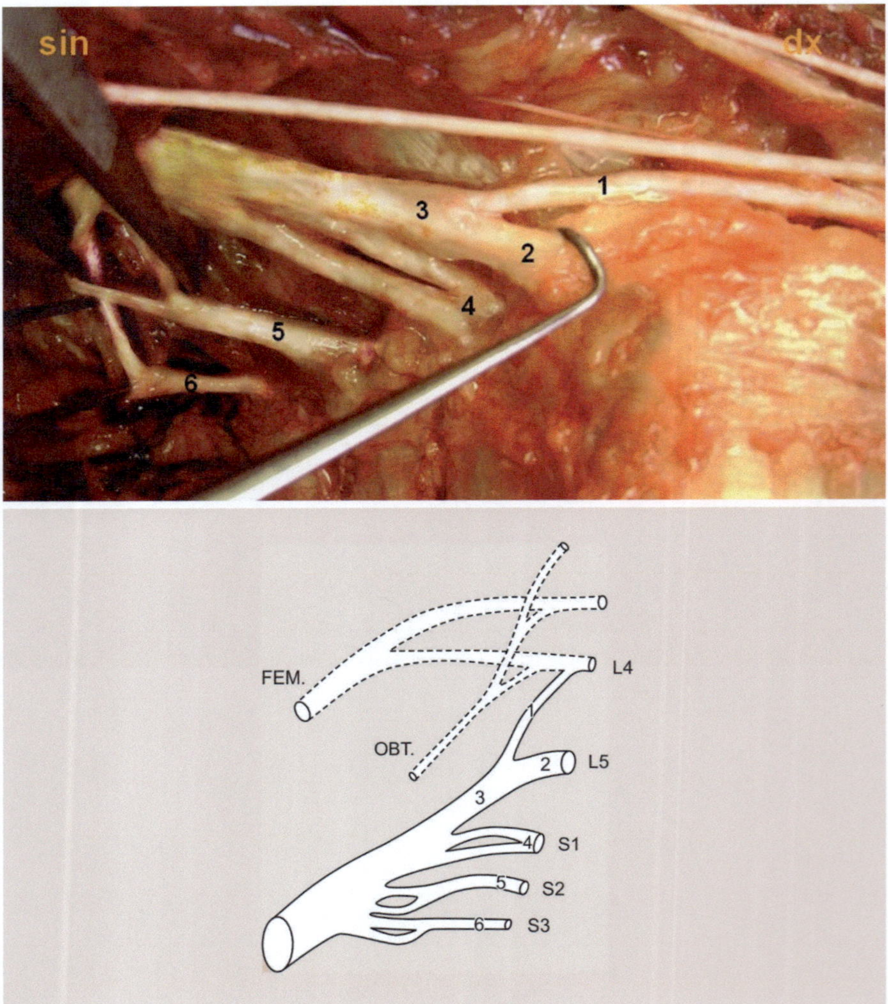

Fig. 8.18 Double root S1, right side. Front view, craniocaudal direction (right to left)—branch from L4 root (1), L5 root (2), lumbosacral trunk (3), S1 root (4), S2 root (5), S3 root (6) (photo captured by Prof. Viktor Matejčík, scheme illustrated by Ms. Anna Francová)

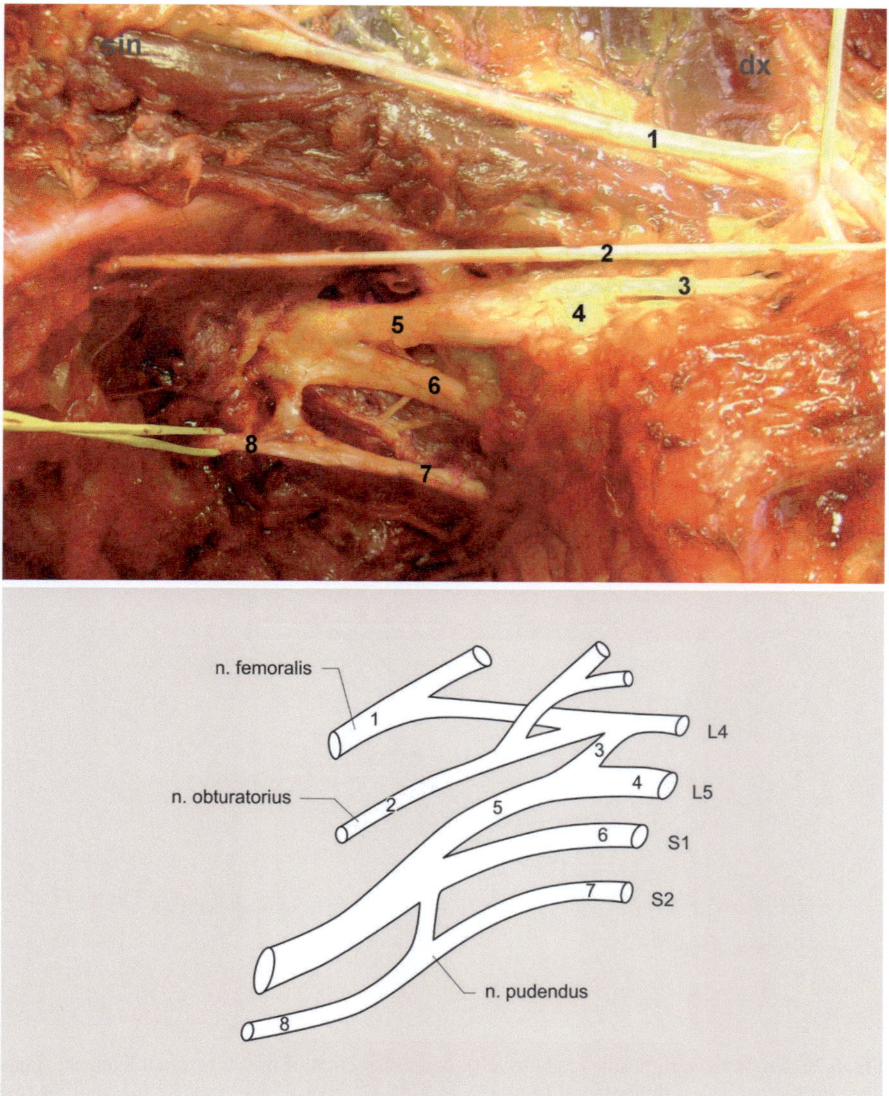

Fig. 8.19 Prefixed type of the lumbosacral plexus. Front view, right side, craniocaudal direction (right to left). In the formation of the pudendal nerve, the S2 root is dominantly involved. Femoral nerve (1), obturator nerve (2), branch from L4 root (3), L5 root (4), lumbosacral trunk (5). S1 root (6), S2 root (7), pudendal nerve (8) (photo captured by Prof. Viktor Matejčík, scheme illustrated by Ms. Anna Francová)

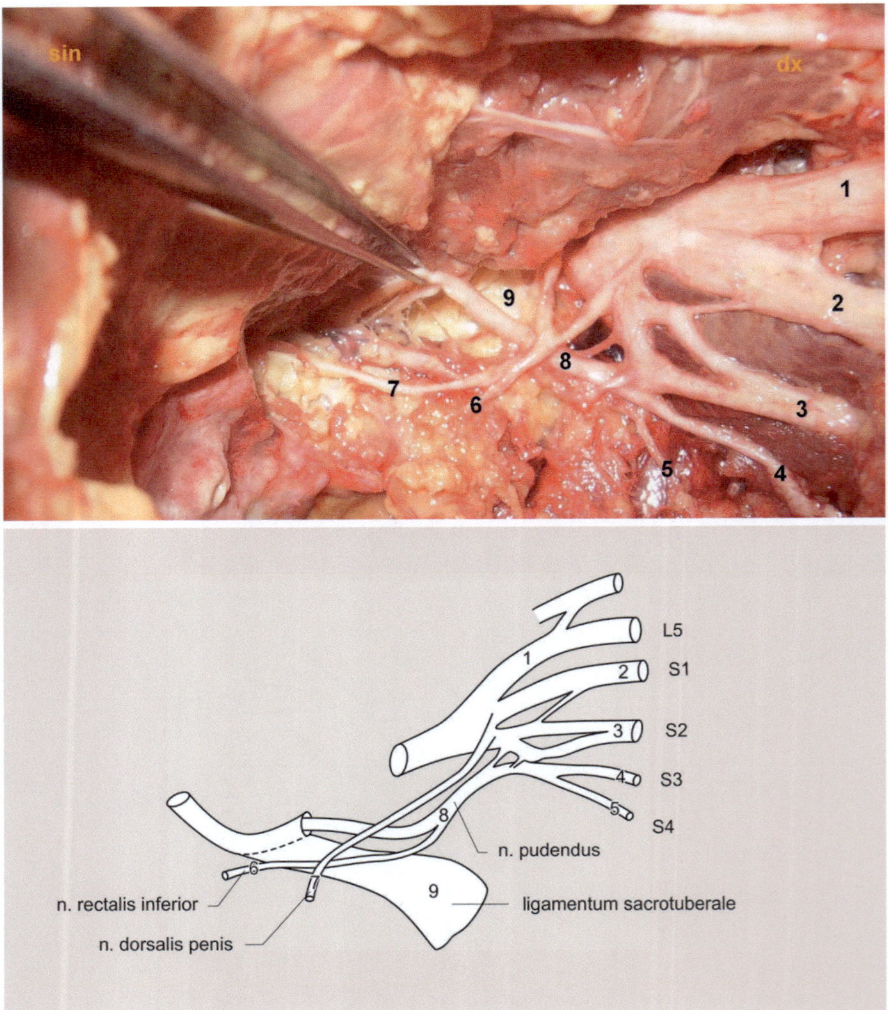

Fig. 8.20 Front view, right side (right to left). After dissection of the sacrospinal ligament (ligamentum sacrospinale): lumbosacral trunk (1), root S1 (2), root S2 (3), root S3 (4), root S4 (5), inferior rectal nerve (n. rectal inferior) (6), dorsal nerve of penis (n. dorsalis penis) (7), pudendal nerve (8), sacrotuberous ligament (ligamentum sacrotuberale) (9) (photo captured by Prof. Viktor Matejčík, scheme illustrated by Mrs. Anna Francová)

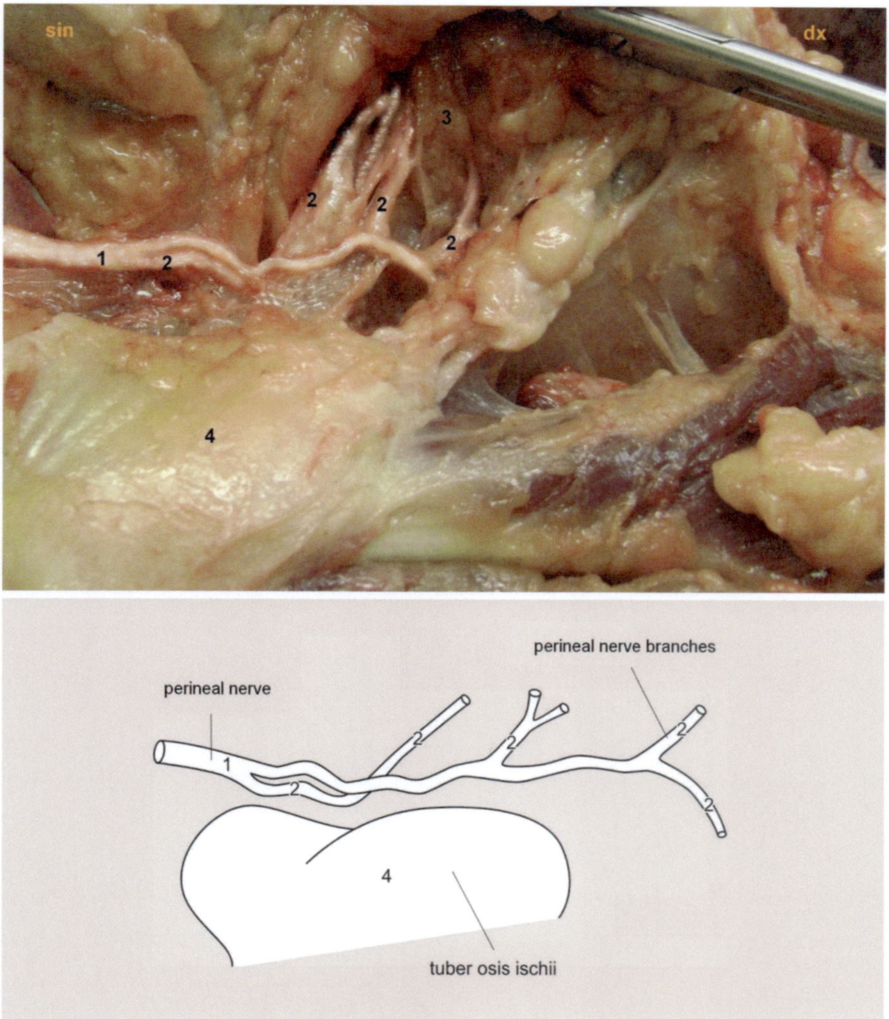

Fig. 8.21 Posterior view, right side (left to right)—perineal nerve (1), branches of the perineal nerve (2), ischiorectal fossa (fossa ischiorectalis) (3), ischial tuberosity (tuber osis ischii) (4) (photo captured by Prof. Viktor Matejčík, scheme illustrated by Ms. Anna Francová)

References

1. Iszi Y, Gürkncar D, Ozan H, Gönül E. The morphological aspects of lumbar plexus and roots. An anatomical study. Turk Neurosurg. 2005;15(2):87–92.
2. Webber RH. Some variations in the lumbar plexus of nerves in man. Acta Anat (Basel). 1961;44:336–45.
3. Erbil KM, Onderoğlu S, Başar R. Unusual branching in lumbar plexus: case report. Folia Morphol (Warsz). 1998;57(4):377–81.
4. Takahashi Y, Sipp D, Enomoto H. Tissue interactions in neural crest cell development and disease. Science. 2013;341(6148):860–3.
5. Šulla I, Balik V, Horňák S, Ledecký V. Cauda equina syndrome in dogs—review. Acta Vet Brno. 2018;87(4):321–33.

Chapter 9
Intraspinal (Extradural and Intradural) Spinal Nerve Variations

Forty-three cadavers were examined as part of the study for this aim. In the prone position of the body, the paravertebral muscles were separated from the spinous processes (processus spinosi) and laminae on both sides from the cervical-cranial (CC) junction to the sacrum. The spinous processes were removed with forceps and a Striker's saw. The laminae on both sides, as well as parts of the articular processes, were removed with a Kerrison. Such "unroofing" of the vertebral canal allowed direct visualization of the spinal cord and nerve roots. A wide laminectomy from the cervical-cranial transition to the sacrum exposed the entire spinal canal to examine each cervical, thoracic, lumbar, and sacral nerve root from its exit from the spinal cord to its exit from the spinal canal through the intervertebral foramen (foramen intervertebrale) and sacral hiatus (hiatus sacralis). Subsequently, a longitudinal dural incision was made to allow direct visualization of the spinal cord, conus medullaris, and spinal nerve roots. The exposed spinal cord segments and nerve roots were examined, observed, and researched, including a detailed examination of their intradural and extradural anastomoses. All intradural and extradural anastomoses were examined for the presence of nerve tissue. During the analysis of intraspinal variations, we also observed the intraspinal formation of the plexuses [1–4]. We defined the plexus type by identification from the C2 root. The intumescences had a different range of shapes and formations [3, 5, 6]. In the prefixed type, they are shorter and more pronounced, and in the postfixed type, they are longer and less pronounced. In the most common type (normotype), at the cranial end of the cervical intumescence, which is at the level of the C5 vertebra, the C6 root recedes. With the prefixed type, it is the C5 root, and with the postfixed type, it is the C7 and C8 (Fig. 9.1, Tables 9.1, 9.2 and 9.3).

The cranial end of the lumbar intumescence is at the level of the T12 vertebra, from which the L3 root departs in the normotype L2 in the prefixed type and L4 and L5 in the postfixed type. Determination of the type of plexus was more reliable when based on the formation of intradural roots. It was not always possible to

Z. Haviarová et al., *Peripheral Nervous System*,
https://doi.org/10.1007/978-3-031-73744-2_9

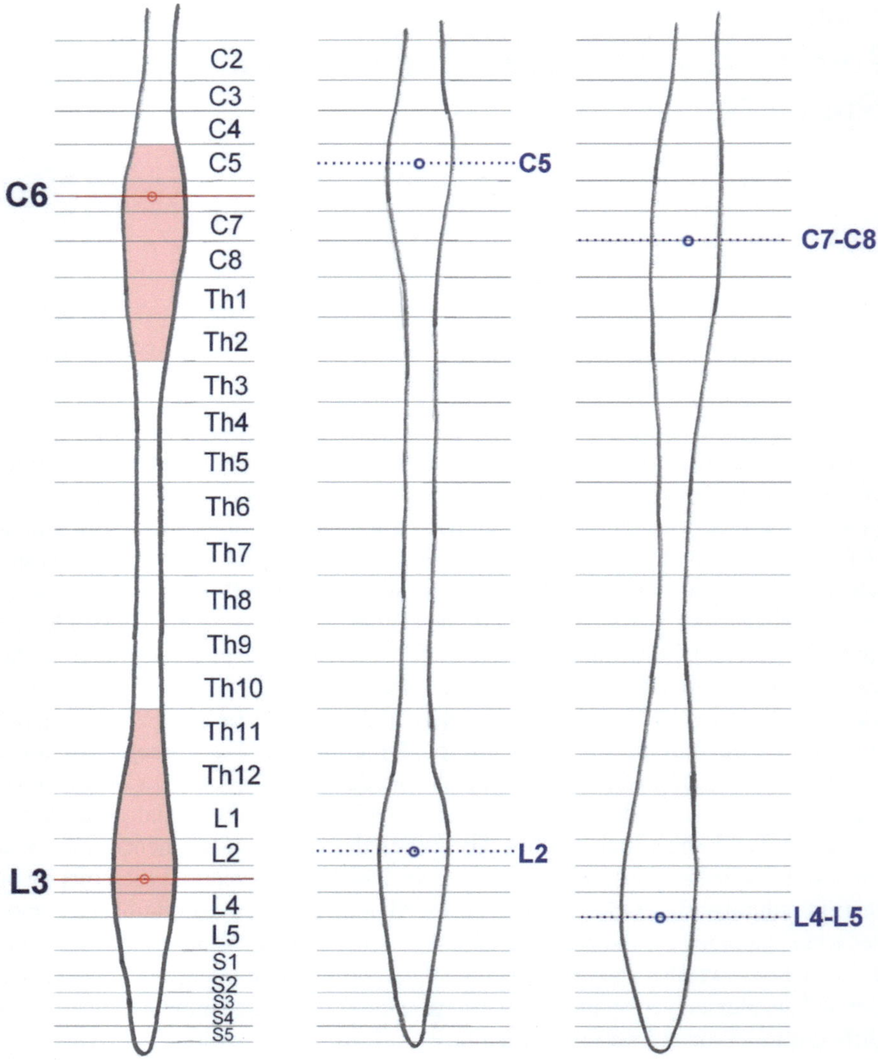

Fig. 9.1 Scheme of normal, prefixed, and postfixed types of plexus (illustrated by Ms. Anna Francová)

clearly define the type of plexus. There was a borderline-transitional type with a tendency toward the prefixed and sometimes postfixed type. Variations were more frequent in the lumbosacral region and were more numerous in the distal direction. Intraspinal intradural variations were observed in all cases of the lumbosacral plexus. In nine cases, it was in the chest area, 20.9% (Tables 9.1, 9.2 and 9.3).

Extradural variations were observed in 60.5% of cases. The distance of the roots in the prefixed type in the lumbar intumescence (intumescentia lumbosacralis) was less obvious. We also observed the merging—assimilation of segments in the distance of the sacral roots. In the prefixed type, the anterior root of L4 is thicker or of

Table 9.1 Atypical spacing—intraspinal intradural variations

Plexus type	Number	Common or close double spacing of roots from one segment			Asymmetry of roots			Missing ventral root			Missing of both ventral and dorsal roots		
		C	*T*	*LS*	*C*	*T*	*LS*	*C*	*T*	*LS*	*C*	*T*	*LS*
Normotype	30	2	2	15	2	1	22	–	–	4	–	–	–
Prefix. type	9	–	–	5	3	1	5	–	–	7	–	–	3
Postfix. type	4	1	–	2	2	1	4	–	–	2	–	–	–
	43	**3**	**2**	**22**	**7**	**3**	**31**	**0**	**0**	**13**	**0**	**0**	**3**

Prefix.—prefixed; *Postfix.*—postfixed; *C*—cervical, bilateral; *T*—thoracic; *LS*—lumbosacral

Table 9.2 Intraspinal intradural variations of nerve roots

Plexus type	Number	Anastomoses between dorsal roots			Anastomoses between ventral roots			Anastomoses between dorsal and ventral roots			Multiple anastomoses		
		C	*T*	*LS*	*C*	*T*	*LS*	*C*	*T*	*LS*	*C*	*T*	*LS*
Normotype	30	12	–	30	1	1	6	1	–	6	6	–	30
Prefix. type	9	3	2	9	1	–	2	–	–	3	1	1	9
Postfix. type	4	2	–	4	–	–	1	1	–	1	–	–	4
	43	**3**	**2**	**22**	**7**	**3**	**31**	**2**	**0**	**10**	**7**	**1**	**43**

Prefix.—prefixed; *Postfix.*—postfixed; *C*—cervical, bilateral; *T*—thoracic; *LS*—lumbosacral

Table 9.3 Intraspinal extradural variations

Plexus type	Number	Atypical spacing of roots			Two roots leading to one neuroforamen			Extradural rami communicantes			Extradural missing nerve root		
		C	*T*	*LS*	*C*	*T*	*LS*	*C*	*T*	*LS*	*C*	*T*	*LS*
Normotype	30	1	2	2	–	2	1	4	1	1	–	–	–
Prefix. Type	9	1	–	–	–	–	–	–	–	1	–	–	3
Postfix. Type	4	1	–	2	1	–	–	1	1	–	–	–	–
	43	**3**	**2**	**4**	**1**	**2**	**1**	**5**	**2**	**2**	**0**	**0**	**3**

Prefix.—prefixed; *Postfix.*—postfixed; *C*—cervical, bilateral; *T*—thoracic; *LS*—lumbosacral

the same thickness as the anterior roots of L5, S1, and S2. The anterior branch of the L3 root was equal in thickness to the anterior branch of the L5 and S1 roots in some cases (11.6%). The lumbar intumescence was more clearly formed with a peak at the level of the L2-L3 diverging roots. With the prefixed and especially postfixed type of plexus, asymmetry of the roots, their atypical distance, multiple anastomoses (especially between the posterior sacral roots) both at a short distance and at a longer distance from the spinal cord, and the absence of a root (in three cases) were more often observed (Table 9.2, Fig. 9.2). In the prefixed type, anastomoses were rare and only between the anterior roots.

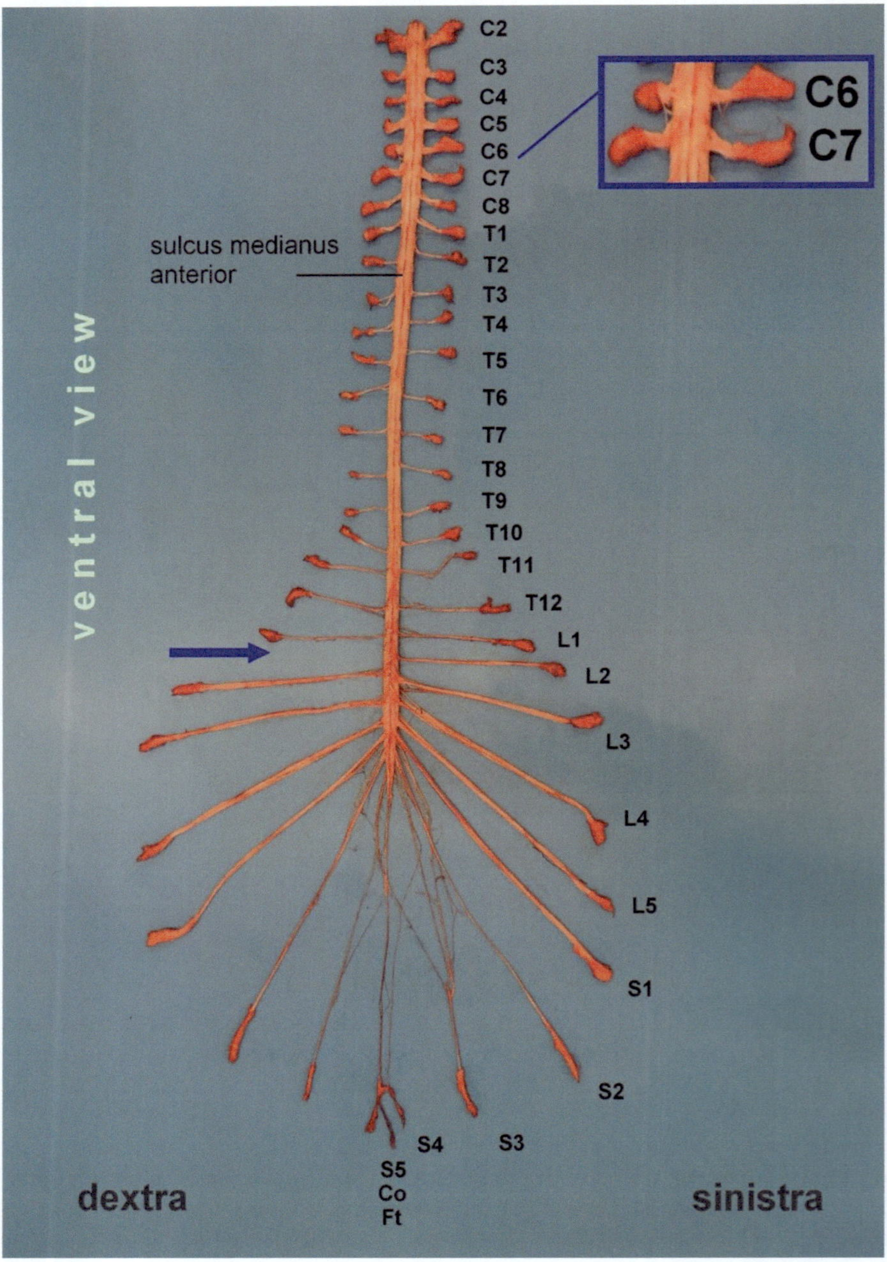

Fig. 9.2 Front view. Anastomosis between the anterior roots of C6 and C7. The root of S2's right side (l. dx) is missing—anastomosis between the dorsal roots of S3's right side (dx.) and S3's left side (sin.) and anastomosis between the dorsal roots of S1 and S2 sin and S1–S3 sin. The L4 and L5 roots are thicker than the S3, S4, and S5 roots (photo captured by Prof. Viktor Matejčík)

In extradural intraspinal variations, an atypical distance of the nerve roots was observed in 20.9% of cases.

Extradural anastomoses between nerve roots were observed in nine cases. In the cervical and especially the lumbar section/region of the spinal cord, from which the nerves of the limbs are formed, connections between the roots are more often possible, since these segments undergo the most significant changes during intrauterine development. It is not only the number of segments that make up the limbs and the nerves that innervate them but also the level of these segments that is important. It is known that the process of moving limbs, accompanied by the "assimilation" of new segments, is of great importance in the formation of plexuses. Anatomical differences testify to the fact that segmentality in the construction of different sections of the human body is not preserved in the same way; it is best preserved in the chest region. In other areas, the segmentality is not so clear. It is especially complicated in the head area and in the areas of the spinal cord that correspond to the levels of limb formation. In the areas of the peripheral nervous system corresponding to the head and limbs—a compartment made up of a large number of segments—we can expect the formation of complex connections. In some areas—regions (face, hand-fist, foot, perianal area)—a combination of three or more segments is observed with a relatively small area [7]. As a result of such multisegmented participation, individual parts of the skin and muscles receive axons from several neurotomes. Thus, the paths of axons to the final territories in the nerves of the head, limbs, and peri-anogenital region acquire great complexity. The junctions that appear in the area of the plexuses and between the nerves of the limbs testify to the complexity of the passage of axons from the assembly of one nerve to the assembly of another, which is associated with the formation of "arches and circular" junctions between the nerves of the limbs. The paths of axons, although unstable, are determined by the segmental origin of nerves.

References

1. Solmaz B, Tatarlı N, Ceylan D, Keleş E, Çavdar S. Intradural communication between dorsal rootlets of spinal nerves: their clinical significance. Acta Neurochir. 2015;157(6):1069–76. discussion 1076
2. O'Rahilly R, Müller F, Meyer DB. The human vertebral column at the end of the embryonic period proper. 4. The sacrococcygeal region. J Anat. 1990;168:95–111.
3. Chotigavanich C, Sawangnatra S. Anomalies of the lumbosacral nerve roots. An anatomic investigation. Clin Orthop Relat Res. 1992;278:46–50.
4. Cahill DR, Leonard RJ. Missteps and masquerade in American medical academe: clinical anatomists call for action. Clin Anat. 1999;12(3):220–2.
5. Tubbs RS, Shoja MM, Loukas M, editors. Bergman's comprehensive encyclopedia of human anatomic variation. Hoboken, NJ: John Wiley & Sons; 2016.
6. Šteňová J, Kubíková E, Šteňo J. Topografické anatomické vzťahy chrbtice, miechy a miechových nervov, význam pre klinickú prax. Neurol pre prax. 2009;10(4):205–8.
7. Lanz T, Wachsmuth W. Kopf: Űbergeordnete systeme, Teil A. Formentwiclung des Kopfes. Teil B. Gehirn- und Augenschädel. Praktische Anatomie, Springer-Verlag. Sonder Ausgabe. 2004.

Part III
Cranial Nerves Variations and Autonomics

Chapter 10
Intracranial Intradural Variations of the Cranial Nerves

The study was performed bilaterally on 60 cadavers. The neurocranium was removed from a horizontal section from the glabella to the inion. After removing the cranial vault, the dura mater was opened, and the cerebrum and cerebellum were bluntly removed from the head. The brain stem was removed. Subsequently, attention was paid to the cranial nerves and the skull base (Tables 10.1, 10.2 and 10.3).

Variations of the abducent nerve (n. abducens) were observed in 48 cases (80%) and variations of the hypoglossal nerve (n. hypoglossus)—atypical origin—in 17 cases (28.3%) (Figs. 10.1, 10.2, 10.3, 10.4, 10.5, 10.6 and 10.7). In four cases (6.6%), simultaneous variations of the hypoglossal and abducent nerves were observed.

Anastomoses between the glossopharyngeal (n. glossopharyngeus) and vagus (n. vagus) nerves were present in four cases (6.6%). Variations of other cranial nerves are extremely rare and described in the literature only as case reports [1–3].

Table 10.1 Intracranial intradural variations of abducens nerve

Total number	**Number of variations**	Double spacing	Bilateral double spacing	Triple spacing	Bilateral triple spacing	Coincidental occurrence of double and triple spacing	Absence of the abducens nerve roots
60	**48**	25	8	5	4	5	1

Table 10.2 Atypical exit of the abducens nerve from the fossa cranium posterior

Total number	Double abducens nerve trunk exit through two foramina	Bilateral double abducens nerve trunk through two foramina	More than double abducens nerve trunk exit through one foramen
5	2	2	1

Z. Haviarová et al., *Peripheral Nervous System*,
https://doi.org/10.1007/978-3-031-73744-2_10

Table 10.3 Atypical exit of the hypoglossal nerve from the fossa cranium posterior

Total number	Bilateral exit double hypoglossal nerve trunk through two foramina	Coincidental occurrence of atypical exit of the double abducens and double hypoglossal nerve through two foramina
17	13	4

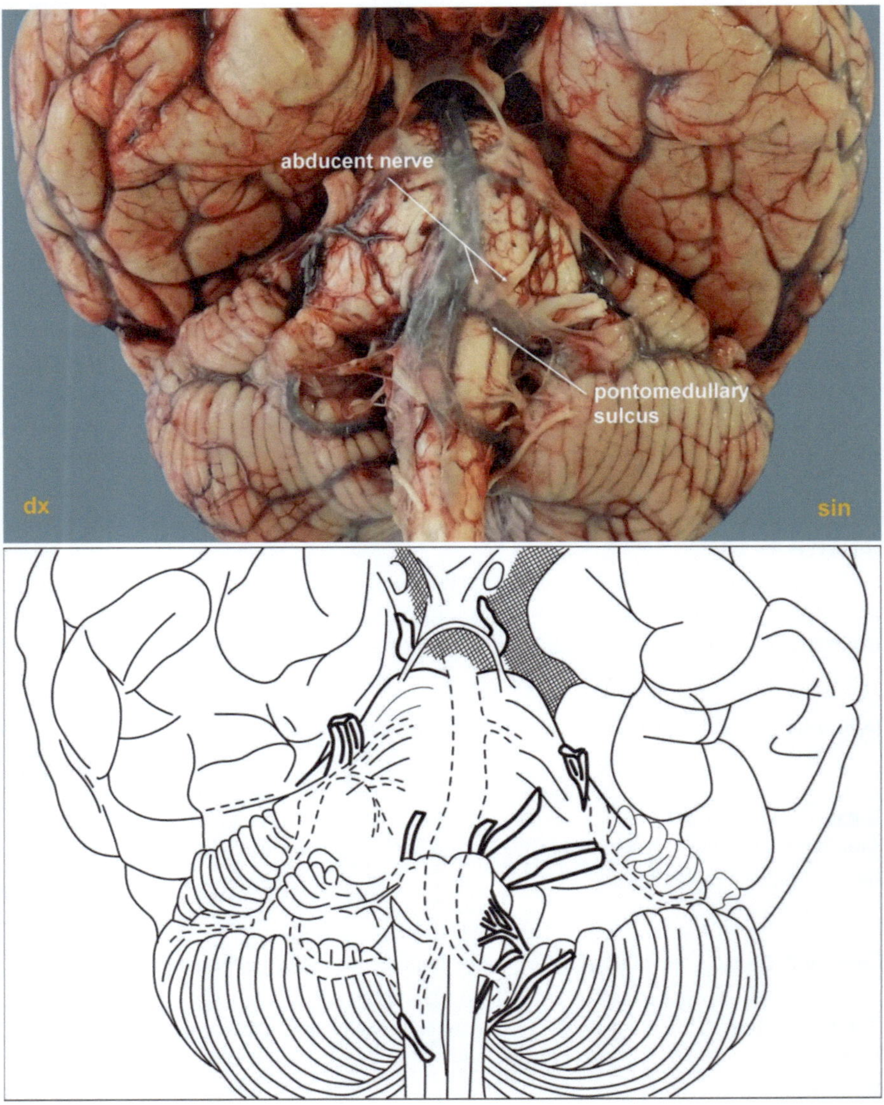

Fig. 10.1 Intracranial intradural variations of cranial nerves: abducens nerve (n. abducens) and hypoglossal nerve (n. hypoglossus). Double spacing of the left abducens nerve (n. abducens l. sin) in the pontomedullary sulcus (photo captured by Prof. Viktor Matejčík, scheme illustrated by Ms. Anna Francová)

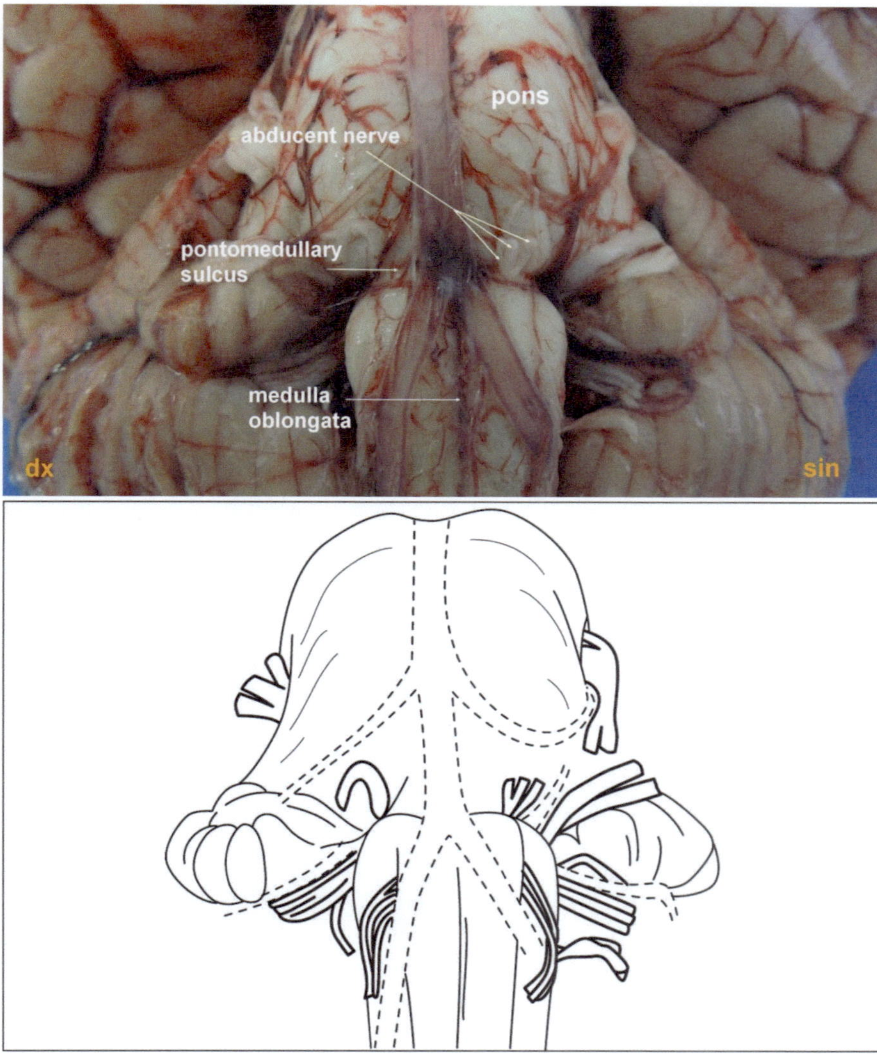

Fig. 10.2 Triple spacing of the left abducens nerve (n. abducens l. sin.) in the pontomedullary sulcus (photo captured by Prof. Viktor Matejčík, scheme illustrated by Ms. Anna Francová)

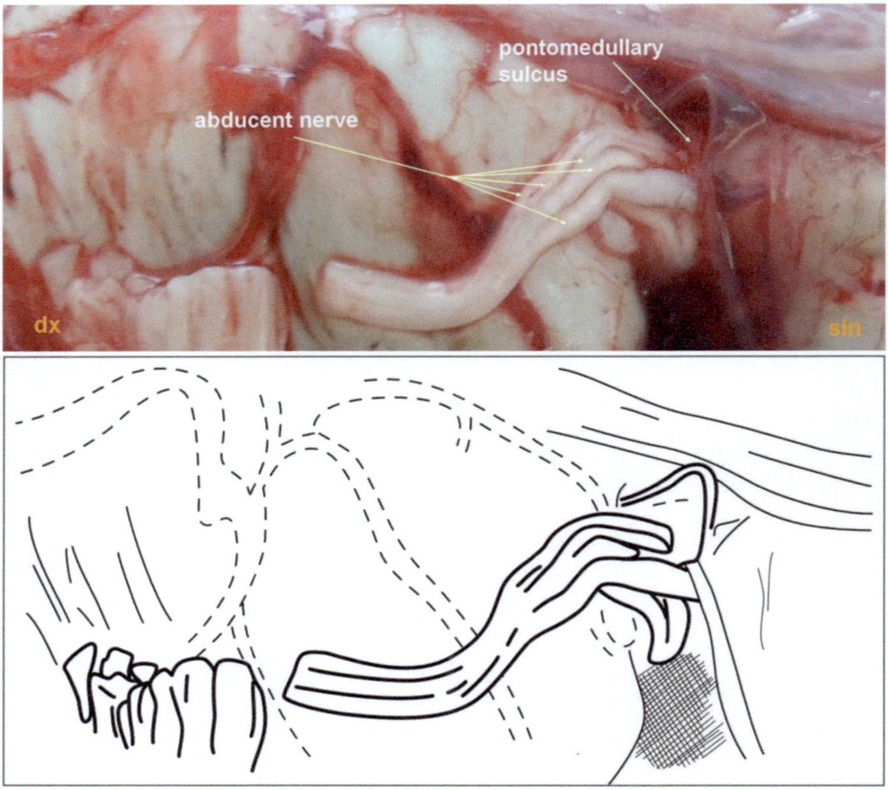

Fig. 10.3 More than three times the distance of the abducens nerve from the pontomedullary sulcus (photo captured by Prof. Viktor Matejčík, scheme illustrated by Ms. Anna Francová)

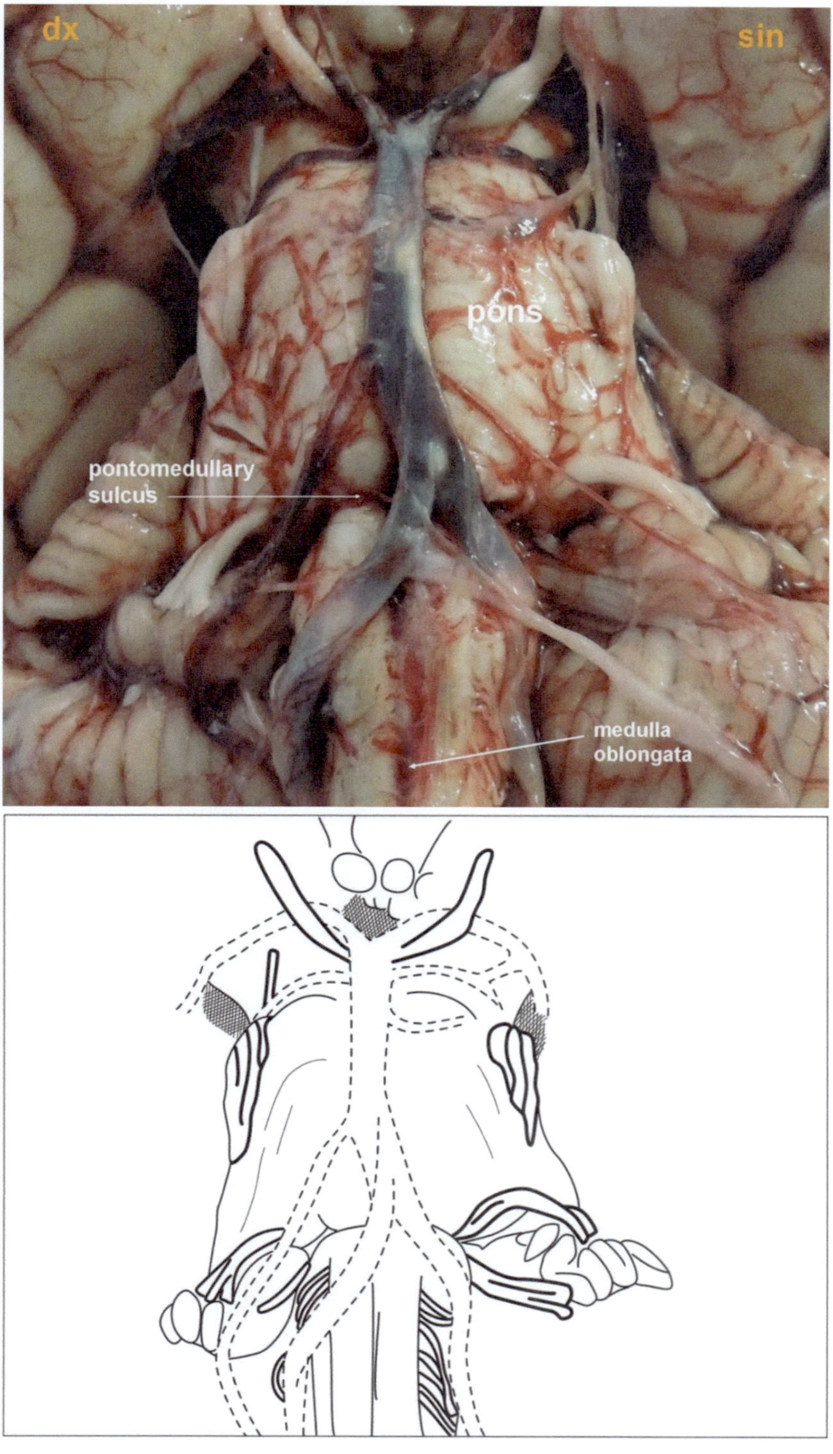

Fig. 10.4 Pontomedullary sulcus. Front view, absence of the abducens nerve (photo captured by Prof. Viktor Matejčík, scheme illustrated by Ms. Anna Francová)

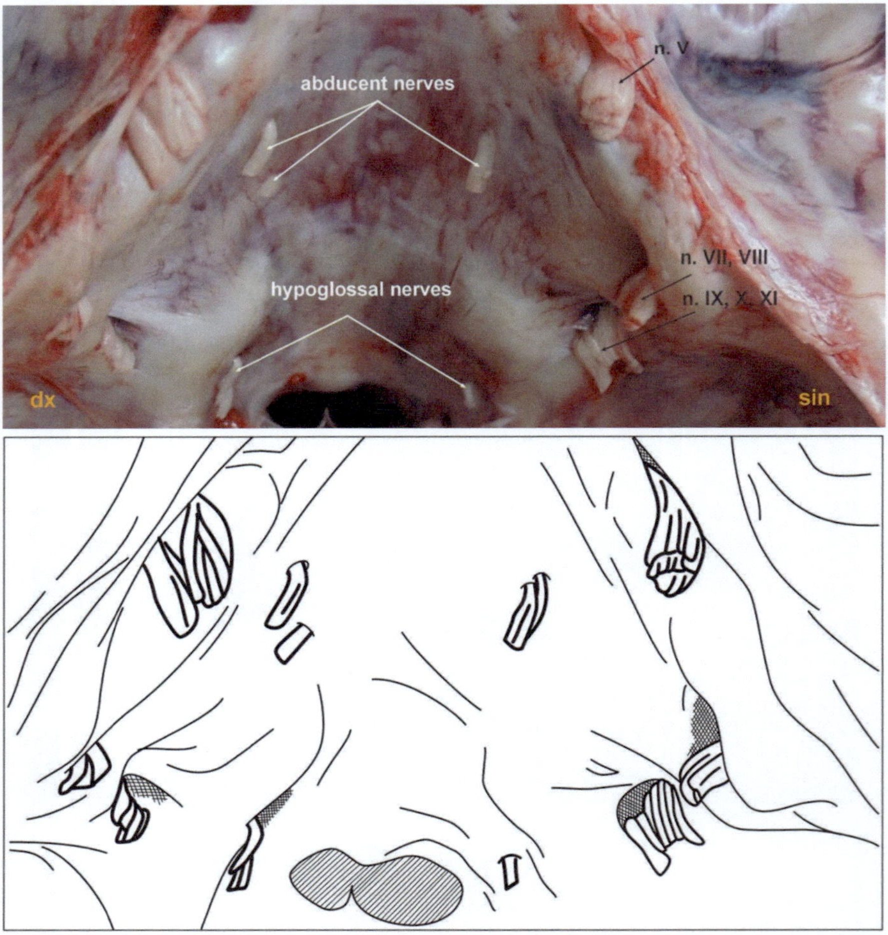

Fig. 10.5 The double exit of the abducens nerve and hypoglossal nerve from the posterior cranial fossa (fossa cranii posterior) through two foramina (photo captured by Prof. Viktor Matejčík, scheme illustrated by Ms. Anna Francová)

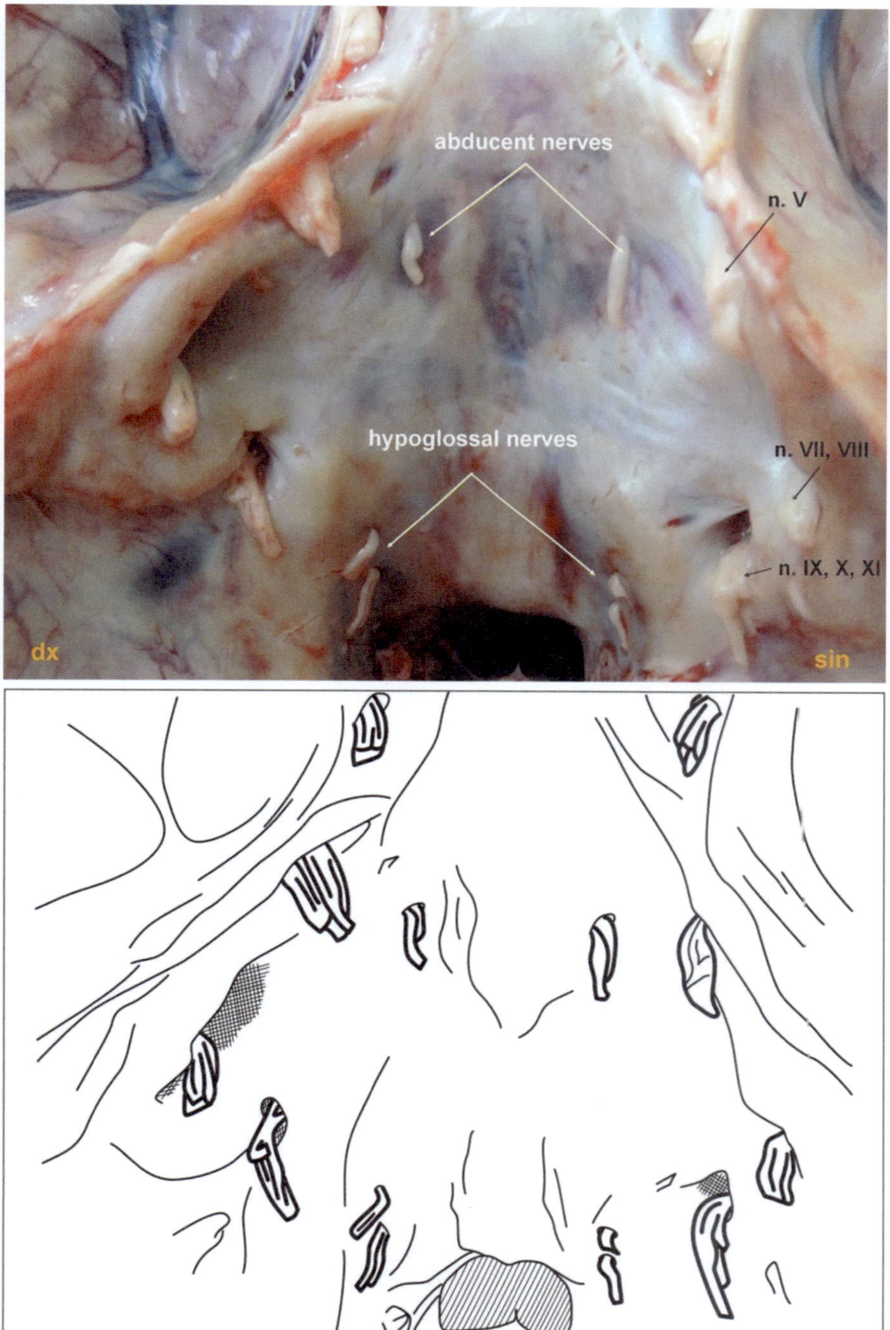

Fig. 10.6 The double exit of the abducens and hypoglossal nerves from the posterior cranial fossa through two foramina (photo captured by Prof. Viktor Matejčík, scheme illustrated by Ms. Anna Francová)

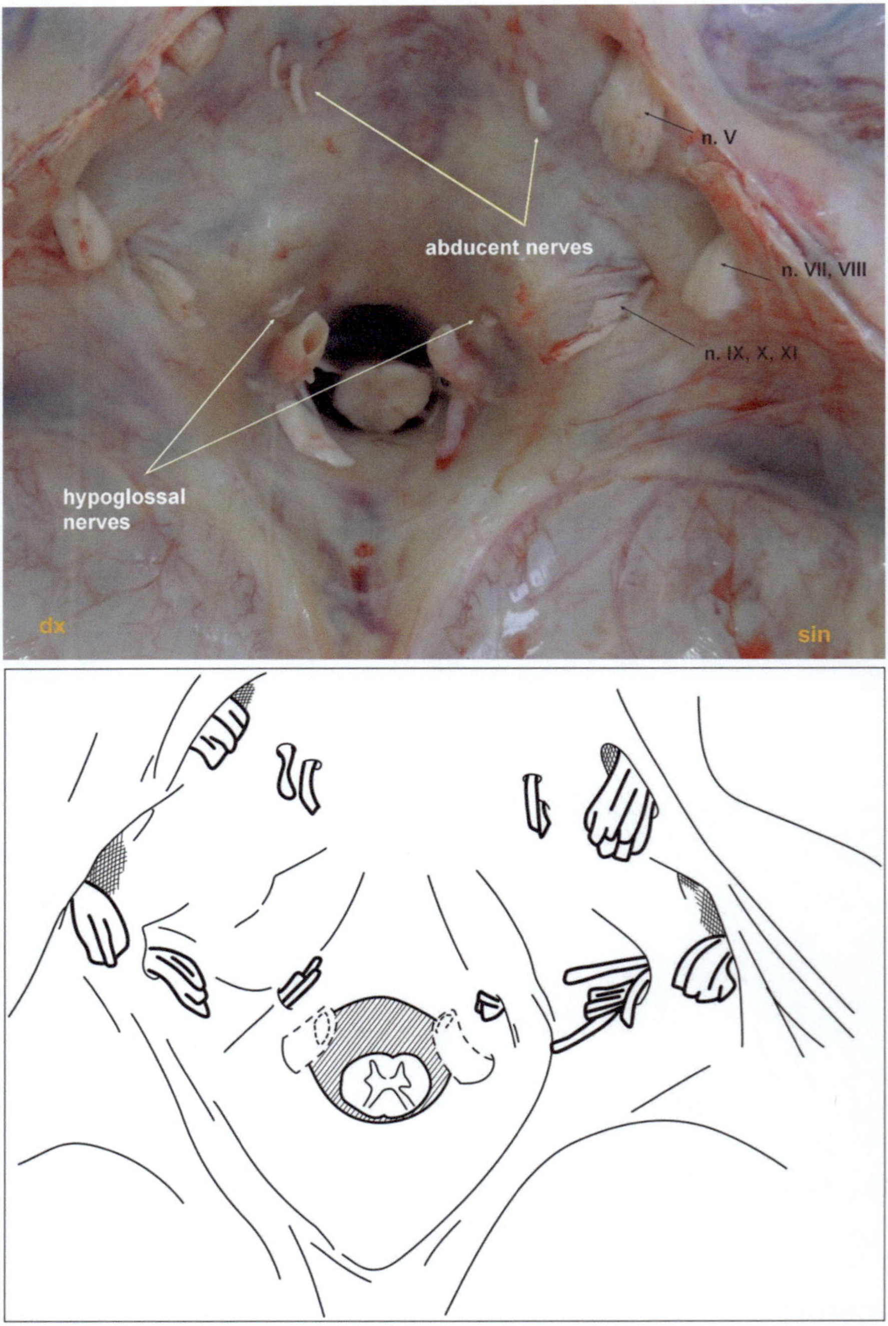

Fig. 10.7 The double exit of the abducens and hypoglossal nerves from the posterior cranial fossa through two foramina (photo captured by Prof. Viktor Matejčík, scheme illustrated by Ms. Anna Francová)

References

1. Coquet T, Lefranc M, Chenin L, Foulon P, Havet É, Peltier J. Unilateral duplicated abducens nerve coursing through both the sphenopetroclival venous gulf and cavernous sinus: a case report. Surg Radiol Anat. 2018;40(7):835–40. Erratum in: Surg Radiol Anat. 2018; 40 (11): 1327
2. Ipsalali HO, Ciftci AC, Kilic D, Sendemir G, Seyhan S, Kaya I, Ortug G. Variations of the 6th cranial nerve (nervus abducens) in the petroclival region: a microsurgical study. Morphologie. 2019;103(341 Pt 2):103–9.
3. Joo W, Yoshioka F, Funaki T, Rhoton JR. Microsurgical anatomy of the abducens nerve. Clin Anat. 2012;25(8):1030–42.

Chapter 11
The Autonomic Ganglia of the Cranial Nerves

The study was carried out during the dissection of 20 cadavers. The parasympathetic ganglia of the head are located in the orbit, infratemporal fossa (fossa infratemporalis, ITF), and pterygopalatine fossa (fossa pterygopalatine, PPF). There are three parasympathetic ganglia located in the cranial part of the parasympathetic nervous system [1–4]. They are ciliary, otic, and pterygopalatine ganglia—ganglion ciliare, oticum, and pterygopalatinum (Fig. 11.1). We did not include the fourth parasympathetic submandibular ganglion in our study. The three mentioned parasympathetic ganglia receive preganglionic fibres via the oculomotor nerve (n. oculomotorius, CN III), facial nerve (n. facialis, CN VII), and glossopharyngeal nerve (n. glossopharyngeus, CN IX). Sympathetic and sensory fibres also enter the ganglia but do not form synapses in it.

The neurovascular relations of each ganglion were examined bilaterally. The orbital area was approached through the anterior cranial fossa. After removing the cerebral hemispheres, the orbital ceiling (greater wing of the sphenoid bone and zygomatic bone), the periorbital and retrobulbar fat, and the nerve structures were gradually examined. The ciliary ganglion (CG) was revealed after pushing away the neurovascular structures and lateral rectus muscle of the eyeball (m. rectus lateralis bulbi oculi).

It appeared as an irregular, flattened, star-shaped structure approximately 2 mm in size, surrounded by retrobulbar fat near the orbital apex. In all cases, it was located inferolateral to the optic nerve and the lateral rectus muscle of the eyeball (m. rectus lateralis bulbi oculi). The CG was superimposed on the superior ophthalmic vein (vena ophtalmica superior) and the ophthalmic artery (arteria ophthalmica). In three cases, the ganglion had an oval shape. We did not see the accessory ciliary ganglion in the orbit.

The otic ganglion (ganglion oticum, OG) was exposed by pushing the main trunk of the mandibular nerve (n. mandibularis) upward and backward for better visualization of all three ganglionic roots. The otic ganglion is small, slightly oval, and flat with a size of about 1–2 mm. In four cases, it had an irregular shape like a "lentil".

Z. Haviarová et al., *Peripheral Nervous System*,
https://doi.org/10.1007/978-3-031-73744-2_11

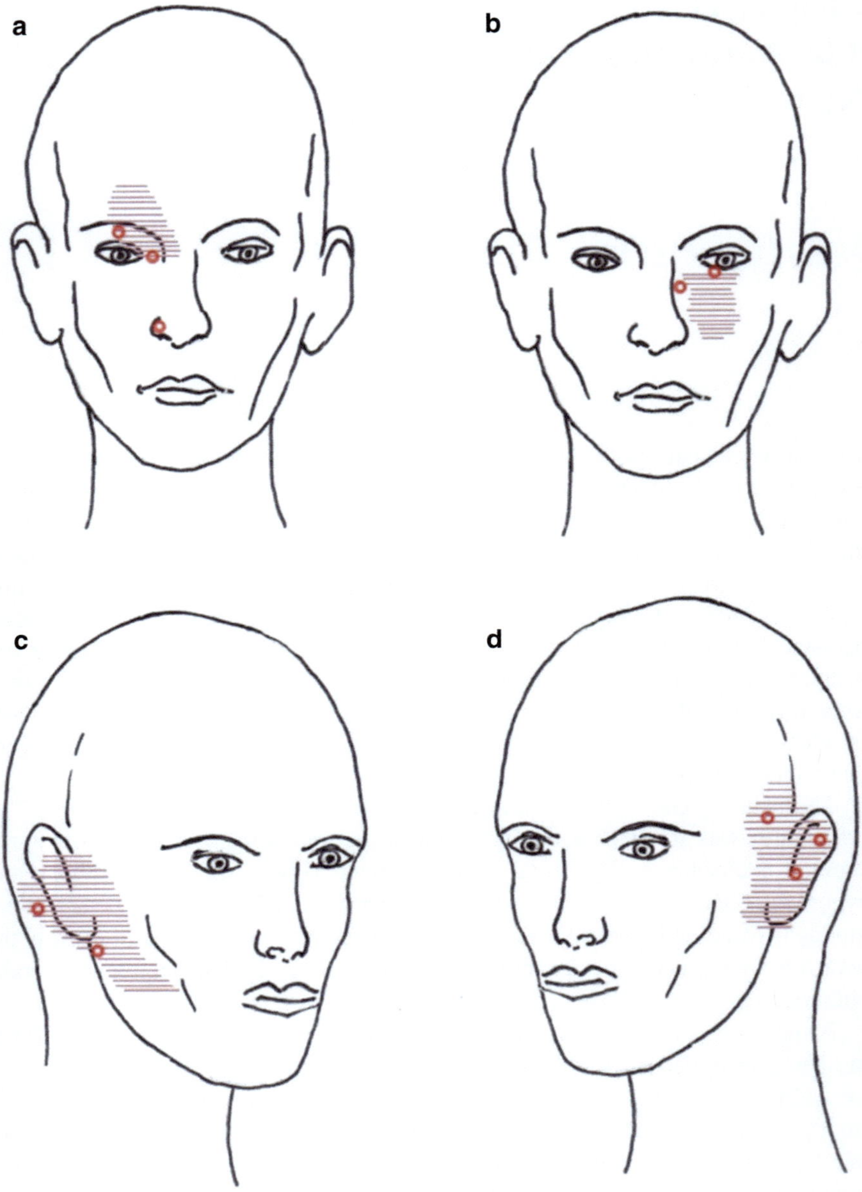

Fig. 11.1 Painful places and areas of their spread in a lesion of the autonomic ganglia of the head. (**a**) damage to the ciliary ganglion, (**b**) damage to the pterygopalatine ganglion, (**c**) damage to the otic ganglion, (**d**) damage to the geniculate ganglion. (illustrated by Ms. Anna Francová)

It was located deep in the ITF just below the oval foramen (foramen ovale), medial to the mandibular nerve (n. mandibularis).

PPG was exposed after the removal of the greater wing of the sphenoid bone (ala major ossis shenoidei). After removing the roof of the PPF, the neurovascular structures and the pterygopalatine ganglion (PPG) located inside this space had a triangular or conical shape. In six cases (30%), it was flat and had a triangular shape. It was situated under the maxillar nerve (n. maxillaris) inside the PPF, opposite the sphenopalatine foramen (foramen sphenopalatinum) and in front of the pterygoid canal (canalis pterygoideus).

The variability of the autonomic ganglia of the cranial nerves can cause the failure of the treatment of some types of neuralgia; unexpected findings in neurosurgery, dentistry, and dental surgery; and atypical manifestations after injection, in case of blockade of nerves and ganglia.

We did not observe side (right-left) asymmetry and variations between the corresponding ganglia nor regarding their localization, topography, morphology, and configuration of their roots. Neurovascular structures, which are in hard-to-reach areas of the head, are often the objects of pathologic processes, traumas, and other local or systemic diseases, such as "cluster" headaches, migraines, and facial pain syndromes.

Painful zones and areas of their spread in case of a lesion along the autonomic ganglia of the head are as follows: A. the ciliary ganglion (ganglion ciliare), B. the pterygopalatine ganglion (ganglion pterygopalatinum), C. the otic ganglion (ganglion oticum), and D. the geniculate ganglion (ganglion geniculatum) (Fig. 11.1).

Headaches and facial pain syndromes occur in the distribution of the trigeminal nerve (n. trigeminus, CN V.). The mandibular nerve (n. mandibularis, CNV/3) has an additional motor component that runs in a separate fascial compartment via the ITF. Unwanted intravascular injection during the blockade of the inferior alveolar nerve (n. alveolaris inferior) can result in distant complications affecting structures such as the middle ear and eyes. It can lead to paralysis of the branch of the oculomotor nerve (n. oculomotorius), CN III. The total sympathetic block is used for the combined blockade of the stellate (ganglion stellatum) and pterygopalatine (ganglion pterygopalatinum) ganglia in the treatment of postherpetic neuralgia, and it includes the ophthalmic branch of the trigeminal nerve. The pterygopalatine ganglion plays an important role in maintaining intraocular pressure and controlling cerebral vasodilation, which may be associated with headaches of vascular origin.

Parasympathetic ganglia can be damaged in most cases during surgical procedures in the places where they are located. The ciliary ganglion can be damaged by bone fragments and during operations using lateral access to the orbit.

The patient should be informed before the surgical procedure about the possibility of developing mydriatic or tonic pupils as a possible complication. The ciliary ganglion can exceptionally be located on the optic nerve (CN II), which can complicate intraorbital procedures (Fig. 11.2).

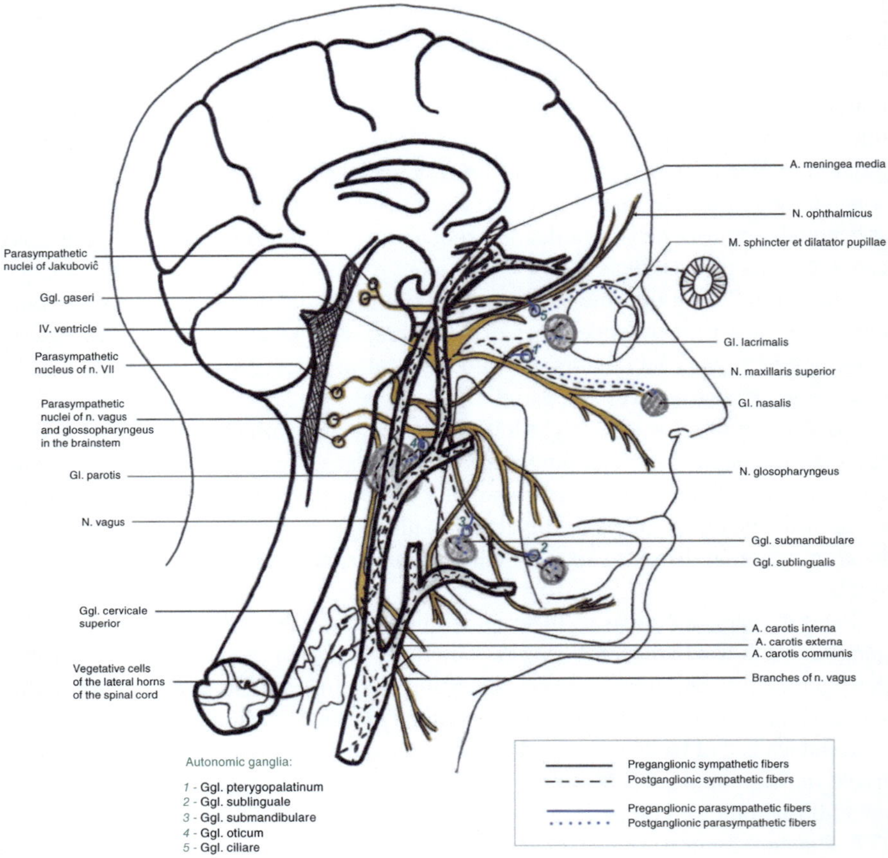

Fig. 11.2 Sympathetic and parasympathetic innervation of the autonomic ganglia of the head (illustrated by Ms. Anna Francová)

The sympathetic nerves also enter the orbit via the first (ophthalmic) and second (maxillary) branches of the trigeminal nerve, not only through the plexus surrounding the ophthalmic artery [5]. Perivascular nerves continue into the lacrimal gland as the lacrimal branches. They may also include parasympathetic fibres from the otic ganglion [6, 7]. Regarding the localization of the three cranial parasympathetic ganglia presented here, our results agree with observations appearing in the literature.

References

1. Siéssere S, Vitti M, Sousa LG, Semprini M, Iyomasa MM, Regalo SC. Anatomic variation of cranial parasympathetic ganglia. Braz Oral Res. 2008;22(2):101–5.
2. Kahle W, Frotscher M. Color atlas and textbook of human anatomy. Volume 3: nervous system and sensory organs. 5th ed. Stuttgart: Thieme Verlag; 2002.
3. Tubbs RS, Menendez J, Loukas M, Shoja MM, Shokouhi G, Salter EG, Cohen-Gadol A. The petrosal nerves: anatomy, pathology, and surgical considerations. Clin Anat. 2009;22(5):537–44.
4. Tubbs RS, Custis JW, Salter EG, Sheetz J, Zehren SJ, Oakes WJ. Landmarks for the greater petrosal nerve. Clin Anat. 2005;18(3):210–4.
5. Thakker MM, Huang J, Possin DE, Ahmadi AJ, Mudumbai R, Orcutt JC, Tarbet KJ, Sires BS. Human orbital sympathetic nerve pathways. Ophthalmic Plast Reconstr Surg. 2008;24(5):360–6.
6. Ruskell GL. Distribution of pterygopalatine ganglion efferents to the lacrimal gland in man. Exp Eye Res. 2004;78(3):329–35.
7. Zhang Y, Liu H, Liu EZ, Lin YZ, Zhao SG, Jing GH. Microsurgical anatomy of the ocular motor nerves. Surg Radiol Anat. 2010;32(7):623–8.

Part IV
Vascular Innervation

Chapter 12
Sources of Nerve Supply to the Vessels of the Extremities and Peculiarities of the Deep Vessels of the Lower Limb Innervation

The clinical observations in patients with complete anatomical interruption of the spinal nerves of the limbs show that these injuries are accompanied by vasomotor disorders [1] and therefore speak of the fact that vascular nerves (nn. vasorum) pass to the final sections in the configuration of spinal nerves. When studying the innervation of vessels, we encounter several questions:

1. In which spinal nerves do the vascular nerves (nn. vasorum) pass, i.e., nerves are the source of the nerve supply of the main vessels?
2. In which section of the vascular trunk is the entry of vascular nerves (nn. vasorum) into the vascular wall most often observed, and what are the sections of the proliferation of the vascular nerves (nn. vasorum) in the vessel walls?
3. What is the relationship of the vascular nerves to the muscular, supraosseus, bone, and articular branches of the basic nerves of the limbs?

All these questions can be solved under the conditions of understanding and solving the innervation of vessels, considering the overall character of the structure of peripheral nerves. It is necessary to determine the entire complex of peripheral nerves, in the composition of which the course of axons forming bundles of vascular nerves (nn. vasorum) is possible. To a certain extent, this will allow us to rationalize surgical interventions, the goal of which is the denervation of one or different parts of the vessel. It is known that in the composition of each spinal nerve, there are autonomic fibres that originate directly from the cells of the spinal cord autonomic centres and enter the spinal nerves through the communicating branches (rr. communicantes). Among such fibres are the vasomotor ones, which leave the spinal nerve trunk in the periphery and form the vascular nerves (nn. vasorum). Thin branches exit from the spinal nerve at various levels throughout its course, which pass into the perivascular space and then into the adventitia of the vessels. So all vessels of the limbs are innervated by the branches of the spinal nerves. The vessels of the organs of the abdominal cavity, retroperitoneal space, and partially the pelvis are supplied by branches of the sympathetic plexuses. Sympathetic, spinal, and

Z. Haviarová et al., *Peripheral Nervous System*,
https://doi.org/10.1007/978-3-031-73744-2_12

cranial nerves participate in the innervation of the vessels of the head. All nerves of the limbs can participate in the innervation of their vessels, especially the main (basic) arteries and veins, but the vascular nerves (nn. vasorum) usually go to the deep vessels of the upper limb in the set of branches of the median, ulnar, and musculocutaneous (n. medianus, ulnaris, and musculocutaneus) nerves, more rarely the radial nerve (n. radialis). In the lower limb, vascular nerves can also accompany all nerves, but they are most often in the saphenous (n. saphenous) and sciatic (n. ischiadicus) nerves. The level of separation of vascular nerves is different. We can observe that either the vascular nerves emerge from the high main trunk and gradually divide into their final branches in the vessel wall or several branches emerge from the main trunk penetrating the vascular wall according to the "segmental" type in some sections, sometimes at a small distance from one to the other. In some cases, almost all cutaneous nerves participate in the innervation of the superficial veins of the upper and lower limbs. In other cases, this amount is much smaller. The same applies to deep vessels. Thus, in the upper limb, in some cases, the vascular branches depart from all nerves; in other cases, the vascular nerves go in a set of only two nerves, most often in the median and ulnar nerve (n. medianus et n. ulnaris).

In some cases, the vessels of the lower limb receive nerves not only from the femoral nerve (specifically from the saphenous nerve) and branches of the sciatic nerve but also from the lateral cutaneous femoral, ilioinguinal, obturator nerves, and others. In other cases, they receive nerves only from the femoral nerve (saphenous nerve) and sciatic nerve.

Vascular nerves originate from the trunk at a sharp angle, subsequently at a certain distance from each other, and sometimes, they pass into the perivascular space and penetrate the adventitia of vessels. They can run in a set of thin muscular, articular, supraosseus, and other branches, which can accompany the blood vessels for a considerable distance and sometimes closely fit them.

In the area of the blood vessel, the vascular nerves divide into upper and lower branches, which after a certain distance pass into the perivascular space and subsequently enter the adventitia of arteries and accompanying veins. Sometimes, we can see that the vascular nerves run along the vessels, and individual short "secondary" branches depart from them, penetrating the vessel wall. We observed a connection between the length of the vascular nerves and vessel diameter—larger diameter vessels have much longer nerves.

The vascular nerves spread and distribute unevenly in the vessel wall, and their number is unstable. Among the vascular nerves, anastomoses often occur both in the adventitia of vessels and in the course of the vascular nerves, which is manifested by the formation of "arches" and "circles".

Anastomoses are observed between the vascular nerves arising from one source as well as from other sources. These are essential connections between the main nerves of the limbs. Vascular nerves supply both, arteries and veins, but the number of branches going to the artery significantly exceeds the number of branches going to the veins. Sometimes, we can observe that vascular nerves penetrate the vein wall in the place of its valve. Peculiarities of the structure of vascular nerves often coincide with several sources—extreme types of nerve variation in the limbs. So, for example, when there are many sources of innervation of vessels in the upper limb, we can observe more and fewer anastomoses between the main trunks of its nerves, indicating a slowing down of nerve differentiation in the limb. In similar cases, axons forming vascular nerves probably have a complex path and pass to the periphery from the assembly of one nerve to the assembly of another. A similar picture is also observed on the lower limb. Here, too, with the presence of anastomoses between the main nerves, the number of sources of innervation of vessels is large, and vice versa, when anastomoses between the main trunks are expressed to a lesser degree (they are rarer or completely absent), the number of sources of innervation such as veins and arteries decreases. In one extreme type of vascular innervation variation (in many sources), the area of expansion of the vascular nerves, coming from one of any nerve, is relatively small, while in the presence of overlapping zones and connections between the vascular nerves (in several cases), we can observe similar networks between the branches of vascular nerves from different sources. Connections between vascular nerves in similar cases occur in large numbers and are observed not only in the adventitia of vessels, in the perivascular space, but also at a considerable distance from the vessels, even in the plexuses, which can be observed in the pulping process.

In the second extreme type of variation (few sources), connections between vascular nerves are rarely observed, and the territories of their distribution differ. These facts allow us to conclude that probably many sources of the nerve supply of vessels are the reflection of the slowing down of the differentiation of the nerves of the limbs. As a rule, thin arteries—branches of the vasa nervorum—run with the vascular nerves. The close anatomical connection between nerves and vessels in the boundaries of the neurovascular bundle witnesses the existing unity not only morphologically, but also functionally. Differences in the sources of innervation of the vessels of the limbs can to a certain extent explain the differences in vasomotor disorders when the same nerves are damaged in different people. With many sources of nerve supply, damage to one trunk (nerve) can cause insignificant vasomotor disturbances in terms of the vastness of the territory. And vice versa, in those cases where the vascular nerves go in a set of only two nerves (median and ulnar nerves on the upper limb; femoral—more precisely saphenous nerve—and sciatic nerves on the lower limb), damage to one of them can cause disruption of vascular function over a large area. Determining the nerves in which the vascular nerves run gives to a certain extent the possibility of clarifying the fact that damage to the median nerve, ulnar nerve, and sciatic nerve (and others) is accompanied by more extensive vasomotor disorders. In the case of lesions to the radial nerve and obturator nerve, these disorders are rarely observed. Various sources of the origin of the so-called nervi vasorum (vascular nerves), different territories of their spread, and the presence of overlapping zones determine the possible irradiation of pain in vascular diseases. Therefore, in thrombophlebitis of superficial and deep veins, in the presence of many sources of innervation, pain can spread to an area far away from the localization of the pathological process. In addition, pain in thrombophlebitis can be explained by the involvement of thin branches passing in the perivascular tissue in the inflammatory process. In similar cases, we can observe degeneration processes of the Wallerian type in the cutaneous nerves of the limbs passing near the superficial veins. Spasms caused by irritation of thin vascular nerves can also be observed with mechanical irritation. These facts explain the presence of venous hyperaemia and cyanosis in conduction disorders in the nerves of the limbs, which are accompanied by the atony of the venous wall. These pathological processes are particularly clearly observed in the case of damage to the sciatic nerve. The close interrelationships between nerves and blood vessels in the boundaries of nerve-vascular bundles are clarified/explained by the spread of the pathological process from vessels to nerves as well. Thrombophlebitis can thus be accompanied by neuritis arising based on involving rr. nervorum. Observed in spontaneous gangrene, the pain can be clarified/caused by drawing the nerve into the arterial pathological process. The described data show how important the different participation of vascular nerves is in the development and course of pathological processes and how important it is to know the complex of nerves in which the vascular nerve fibres run.

Extreme Types of Changes in the Innervation of the Deep Vessels of the Lower Limb

The number of spinal nerves, in the composition of which there participate the vascular nerves (nn. vasorum) to deep vessels, is different [2]. In some cases, the deep vessels of the lower limb are innervated from six sources, in others from three.

In many sources, deep vessels are innervated by branches of the femoral nerve—saphenous nerve—tibial nerve, deep peroneal nerve (n. peronei profundus), obturator nerve (n. obturatorii), lateral cutaneous femoral nerve (n. cutaneous femoris laterales), and ilioinguinal nerve (n. ilioinguinalis). With this type, changes in the territories of vascular nerve extensions are not large, and many anastomoses are observed between the main nerves of the lower limb and their branches on the periphery. In addition, there are connections between vascular nerves forming "arches" and "circles", and in some places, there are numerous connections resembling networks. In such cases, the course of axons in the assembly of vascular nerves is complex. Just as the presence of anastomoses between nerves on the periphery testifies to a certain extent to a slowed differentiation of the nerves of the limbs, so we can suspect that the presence of many sources of the nerve supply of deep vessels and overlapping zones between vascular nerves also indicate a slowed differentiation of nerves.

In other cases, when there are few junctions between the main nerves and their branches on the periphery, or these junctions are almost absent, the axons of the vascular nerves go only in the assembly of three nerves: femoral nerve—saphenous nerve—tibial nerve, and deep peroneal nerve (n. peroneus profundus).

Comparing the two extreme types of variations, it is obvious that in both cases, the vascular nerves pass primarily in the set of femoral nerves—saphenous nerve—tibial nerve, and deep peroneal nerve (n. peroneus profundus).

References

1. Nightingale TE, Mehnert U, Kessler TM, Krassioukov AV. Autonomous nervous system dysfunction. Oxford Textbook of Neurorehabilitation; 2020. p. 111.
2. Feigl GC, Schmid M, Zahn PK, González CAA, Litz RJ. The posterior femoral cutaneous nerve contributes significantly to sensory innervation of the lower leg: an anatomical investigation. Br J Anaesth. 2020;124(3):308–13.

Chapter 13
Sources of Innervation of the Upper Limb Superficial and Deep Veins

Sources of Innervation of the Basilic Vein (Vena Basilica) and Cephalic Vein (V. Cephalica)

The sources of innervation of superficial veins on the ventral and medial surfaces of the shoulder and forearm are the medial cutaneous antebrachial nerve (n. cutaneous antebrachii medialis) (1) and the medial cutaneous brachial nerve (n. cutaneous brachii medialis) (2)(1).

In some cases (Fig. 13.1), the number of sources of vascular nerves (nn. vasorum) is large. The vascular fibres innervating the basilic vein (v. basilica) and its branches are part of almost all skin nerves and are branches in the area of the arm from the medial cutaneous brachial nerve (n. cutaneous brachii medialis) (2) and on the forearm from the medial cutaneous antebrachial nerve (n. cutaneous antebrachii medialis) (1). In other cases (Fig. 13.2), the trunk of the basilic vein (v. basilica) was supplied with branches of the medial cutaneous antebrachial nerve (n. cutaneous antebrachii medialis) [1]. A similar picture is observed when only a small number of cutaneous nerves participate in the innervation of all superficial veins. In several cases, a large number of vascular nerve sources are consistent with the network arrangement of superficial veins. Cutaneous nerves closely adhere to the superficial arteries and veins and intertwine with them (Fig. 13.3a, b).

Vascular nerves are rarely long and usually diverge segmentally. In the confluence of veins, nerves come from two branches of the medial cutaneous antebrachial nerve (n. cutaneous antebrachii medialis) (1) (Fig. 13.3a, b).

In the innervation of the superficial veins on the ventral and lateral surface of the upper limb, the superior and inferior lateral cutaneous brachial nerves (n. cutaneous brachii lateralis superior et inferior), posterior cutaneous brachial nerve (n. cutaneous brachii posterior), lateral antebrachial cutaneous nerve (n. cutaneous antebrachia lateralis), superficial branch of the radial nerve (r. superficialis n. radialis), and dorsal branch of the ulnar nerve (r. dorsalis manus n. ulnaris) participate.

Z. Haviarová et al., *Peripheral Nervous System*,
https://doi.org/10.1007/978-3-031-73744-2_13

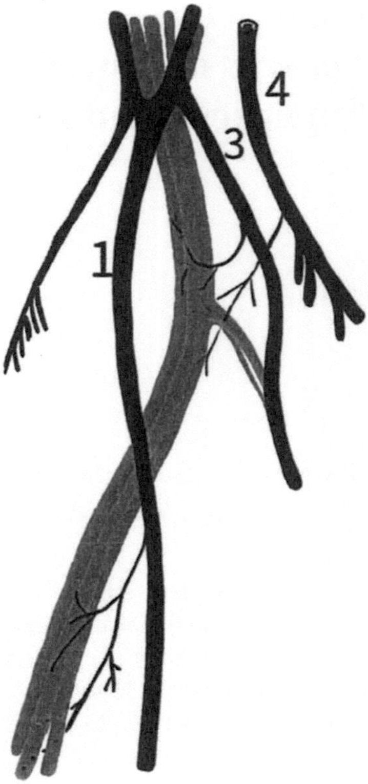

Fig. 13.1 Vascular nerves (nn. vasorum) are part of almost all skin nerves. The basilic vein (v. basilica) and its branches are innervated in the arm from the medial cutaneous brachial nerve (n. cutaneous brachii medialis) (2) and on the forearm from the medial cutaneous antebrachial nerve (n. cutaneous antebrachii medialis) (1) (illustrated by Ms. Anna Francová)

In some cases, more often by the network-like structure of the veins, the aforementioned nerves participate in their innervation.

In other cases, with a small number of anastomoses between the veins, the confluences of cephalic veins (vv. cephalicae) on the forearm are innervated by branches of the lateral cutaneous antebrachial nerve (n. cutaneous antebrachii lateralis) and the superficial branch of the radial nerve (r. superficialis n. radialis). The trunk of the cephalic vein (v. cephalica) is innervated by the recurrent branch of the musculocutaneous nerve (n. musculocutaneous).

In such cases, the complexity of the interrelationships between superficial arteries, veins, and nerves can be observed.

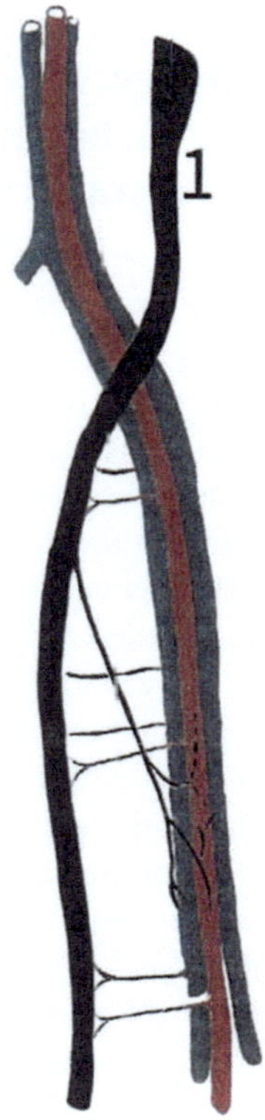

Fig. 13.2 The trunk of the basilic vein is supplied with branches of the medial cutaneous antebrachial nerve (n. cutaneous antebrachii medialis) (1). A similar picture is observed when only a small number of cutaneous nerves participate in the innervation of all superficial veins (illustrated by Ms. Anna Francová)

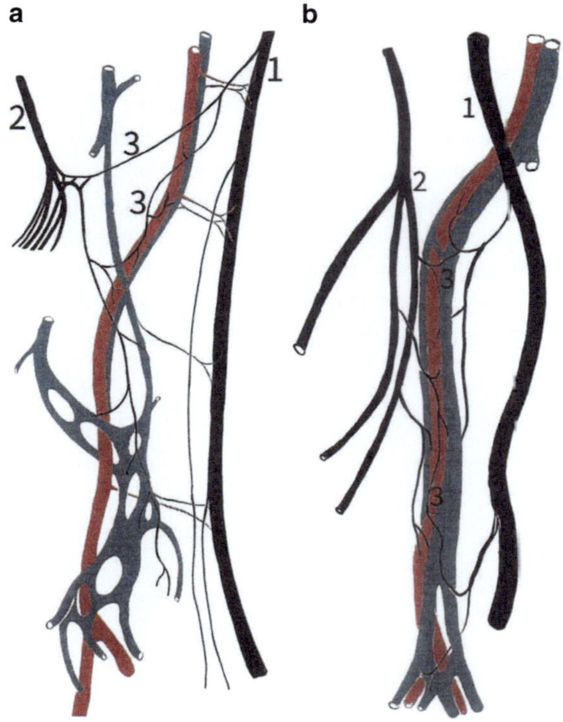

Fig. 13.3 (**a**, **b**) Many vascular nerves are consistent with the network arrangement of superficial veins. Cutaneous nerves closely adjoin and intertwine with superficial arteries and veins. Vascular nerves usually leave segmentally (illustrated by Ms. Anna Francová)

Details of the Interrelationships Between the Sources of Innervation of the Deep Vessels of the Upper Limb and Variations of the Sources of Nerve Supply of the Deep Vessels of the Upper Extremity

In the presence of many sources of vascular nerves, they form arches and circles among themselves. In similar cases, connections between the main trunks are also observed [2].

In some cases, "arcades" are formed in the perivascular space between the vascular nerves, indicating a possible retrograde course of axons. The mentioned data testify to the complexity of the structure of the nerve-vascular bundle. From each nerve belonging to the blood vessels, vascular nerves (nn. vasorum) depart and vice versa from vessels to the nerves of the vasa nervorum.

The veins of the nerve pass along the arteries, while their construction (formation of anastomoses) sometimes coincides with the nature of the connections between vascular nerves and their sources. As a rule, the zones of vascularization of the nerve coincide with the zones of innervation of vessels.

In the innervation of the deep vessels of the upper limb, the median nerve (n. medianus) and the ulnar nerve (n. ulnaris), more rarely the musculocutaneous nerve (n. musculocutaneus) and only exceptionally the radial nerve (n. radialis), take part. In those cases, when all nerves of the upper limb are involved in the innervation of the vessels, we can observe many connections between the main nerves to the periphery. Furthermore, connections between vascular nerves are observed to the same degree, and arches and circuits are formed. The presence of anastomoses between the main nerves indicates a slowed differentiation of the nerves of the limbs, and many sources of innervation of the deep vessels are observed. With slowed nerve differentiation, axons of the vascular nerves (nn. vasorum) reach the periphery via all nerves as their components.

In cases when three nerves participate in the innervation of deep vessels (median nerve, ulnar nerve, and the posterior interosseous nerve of the forearm of the radial nerve (n. interosseus antebrachii posterior)), anastomoses are rarely observed between the main nerves in the periphery and between vascular nerves. The small number of sources of nerve supply to the vessels, as well as the absence of anastomoses between the main nerves, indicates a high degree of differentiation of the peripheral nerves of the upper limb.

References

1. Aliotta RE, Jacob DD, Drake RL, Gurunian L, Gurunian R. Brachial artery and basilic/cephalic veins. Recipient vessels in reconstructive microsurgery: anatomy and technical considerations 2021, 141–148.
2. Sawyer FK, Stefanik JJ, Lufler RS. The branching and innervation pattern of the radial nerve in the forearm: clarifying the literature and understanding variations and their clinical implications. Diagnostics. 2020;10(6):366.

Part V
Lesions of the Innervation of Limb Vessels and Venous Drainage of the Nerves

Chapter 14
Signs of the Spinal Nerve Lesions on the Extremities

In the case of peripheral nerve injury, not only motor and sensory disturbances occur, but also vasomotor disturbances are observed in most cases [1, 2]. The nature and degree of vasomotor disorders differ depending on the individual nerves and the level of their lesion. The difference is also observed in the overall limb external appearance and the appearance of the skin and its colour. In the upper limbs, these differences are particularly pronounced, especially when comparing vasomotor disturbances caused by injury of the radial and median nerves. In the case of lesions of the right median nerve (Fig. 14.1), the colour of the skin, especially the wrist and hand, has a reddish shade (characteristic of arterial hyperaemia), which sometimes turns pinkish red, especially on the palm, and the skin is generally dry, thinned, and slightly shiny.

In case of damage to the radial nerve (Fig. 14.2, left side), the skin, especially the wrist and hand, has a pale blue colour and is slightly thickened and pasty. In addition, in the case of radial nerve, injury is observed as pronounced hypertrichosis on the back of the wrist and hand, as well as on the forearm, although manifestations of hypertrichosis are also observed in injuries of the median nerve, not so often and not so intensively.

In the lower limb, in case of damage to the sciatic nerve, vasomotor disorders are also observed, especially in the foot and ankle (Fig. 14.3). The skin on the back of the instep (tarsus) has a pale blue hue and is thinned and dry to the touch. Trophic disorders are observed mainly on the foot.

Figure 14.4 shows the condition of the axillar and radial nerve injuries in the region of the plexus brachialis. In such cases, the skin of the wrist and hand can have a bluish colour with a hint of purple tint on the dorsal surface of the hand, and swelling, oedema, and pasty hand can be observed. It is caused by the participation of the radial nerve in the innervation of the subcutaneous veins of the forearm and back of the hand. When observing vasomotor disorders and manifestations arising due to peripheral nerve injury, we cannot look at them and consider them as something

Z. Haviarová et al., *Peripheral Nervous System*,
https://doi.org/10.1007/978-3-031-73744-2_14

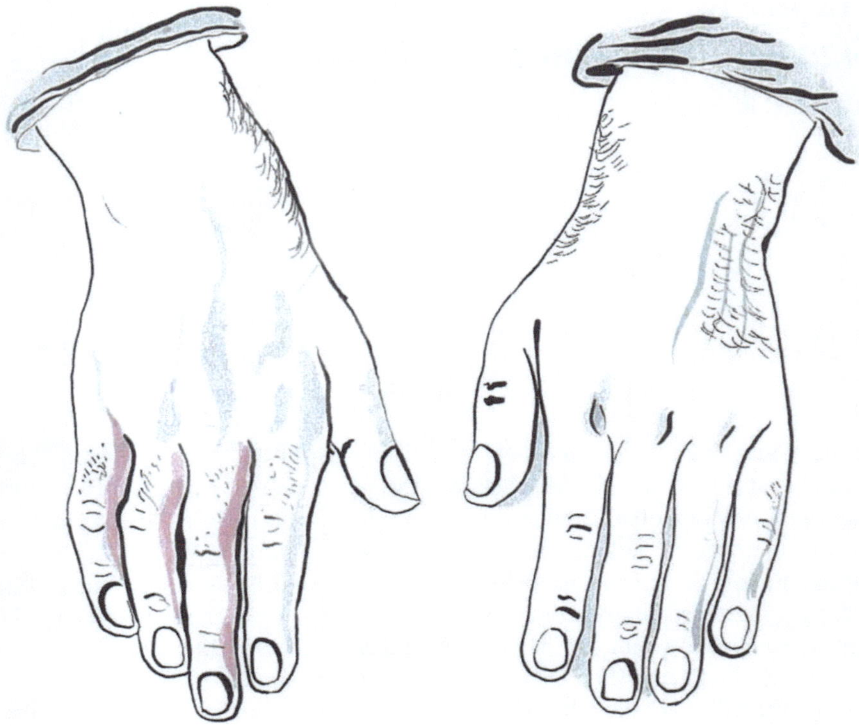

Fig. 14.1 Lesion of the right median nerve (n. medianus l. dx). The colour of the skin, especially the wrist and hand, has a reddish hue (illustrated by Ms. Anna Francová)

isolated—spinal nerves form one complex with neighbouring arteries and veins and in some sections with a dense network, entwining these vessels with sympathetic fibres. Therefore, damage to one of the components of this complicated anatomical structure is accompanied by a series of pathological processes that reflect disturbances of the entire system.

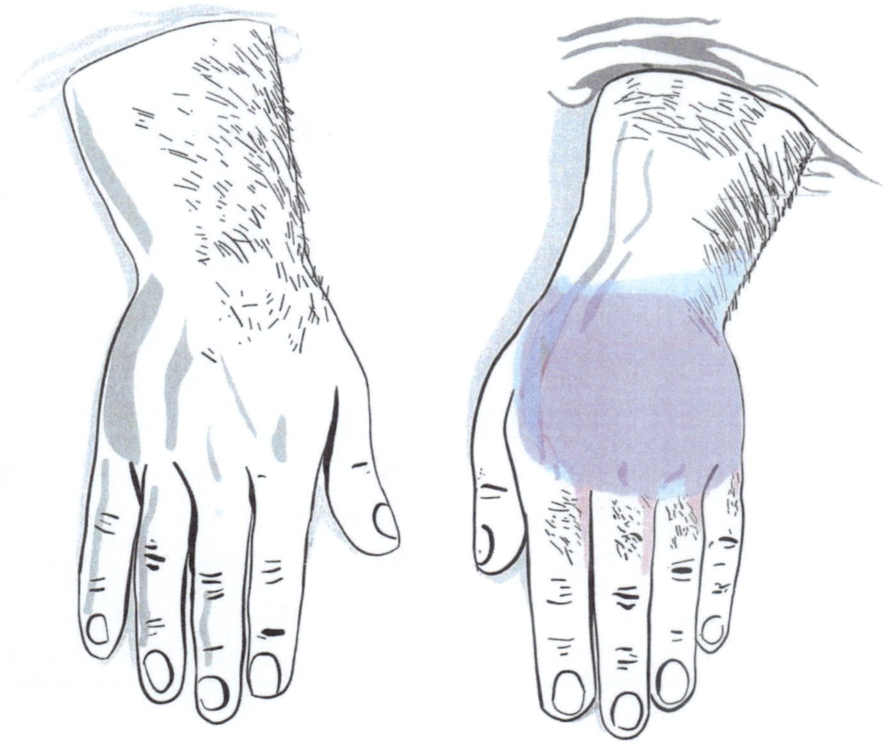

Fig. 14.2 Lesion of the radial nerve. The skin, especially the wrist and hand, has a pale blue colour, the skin is slightly thickened and pasty, and hypertrichosis is observed on the back of the wrist and hand, as well as on the forearm (illustrated by Ms. Anna Francová)

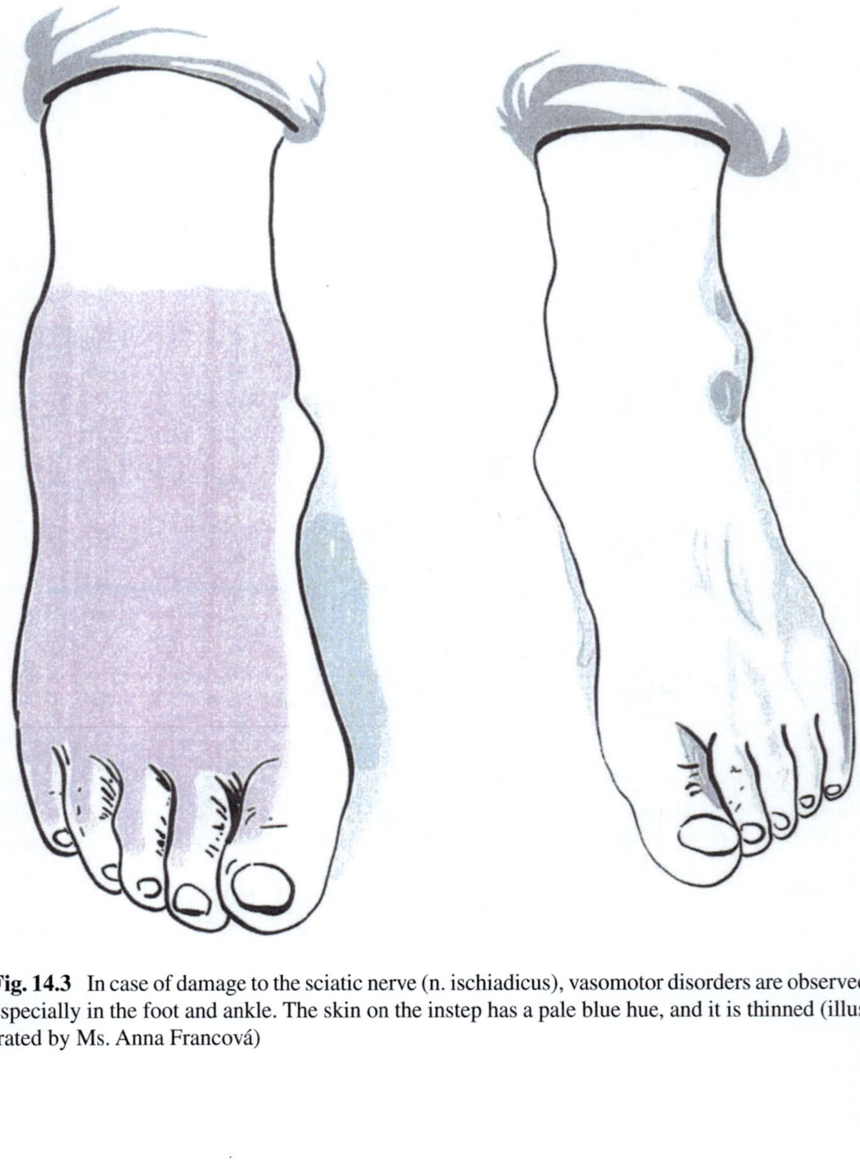

Fig. 14.3 In case of damage to the sciatic nerve (n. ischiadicus), vasomotor disorders are observed, especially in the foot and ankle. The skin on the instep has a pale blue hue, and it is thinned (illustrated by Ms. Anna Francová)

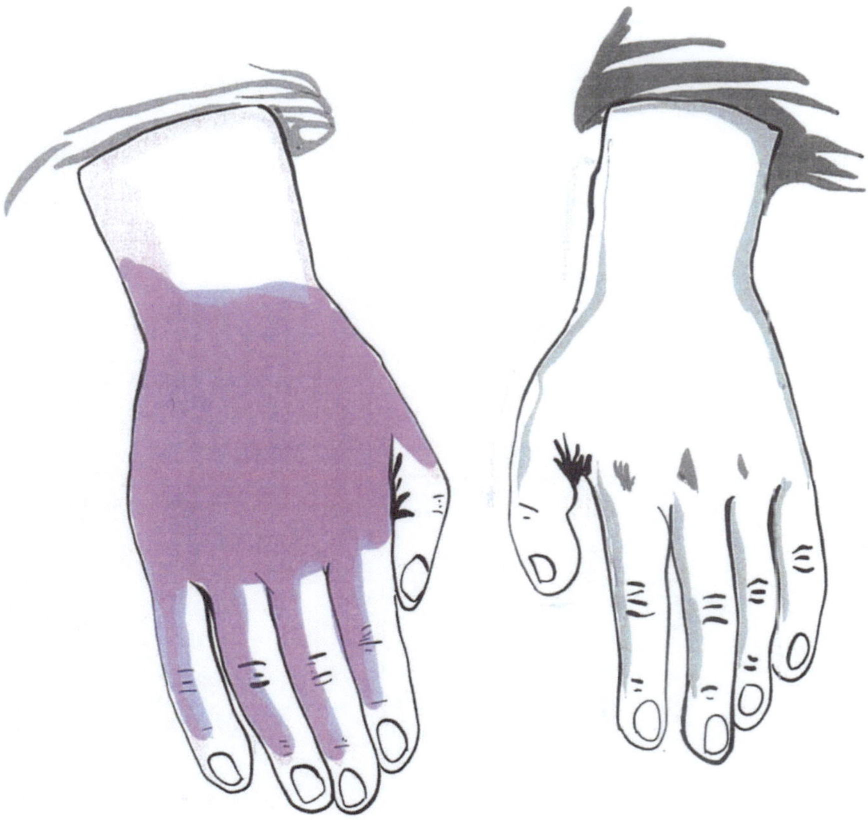

Fig. 14.4 When injured, damage to the axillary and radial nerves in the brachial plexus, the skin of the wrist and the hand may have a bluish colour, and swelling and oedematous pasty hand may be observed (illustrated by Ms. Anna Francová)

References

1. Da Ros V, Picchi E, Ferrazzoli V, Schirinzi T, Sabuzi F, Grillo P, et al. Spinal vascular lesions: anatomy, imaging techniques and treatment. Eur J Radiol Open. 2021;8:100369.
2. Mullins BM, Kelsall N. Anatomy of the lumbar and sacral plexuses and lower limb peripheral neuropathies. Surgery (Oxford). 2023;41(4):193–9.

Chapter 15
Sources of the Nerve Veins

Based on the topography (Fig. 15.1), we distinguish the extratrunkal veins of the nerve (1) and intratrunkal ones. The first occurs in the paraneural space and the second in the nerve sheaths. In connection with this, we distinguish epineural (2), perineural (3), and endoneural veins (4). The largest of them are usually located in the part of the nerve facing the vessels running in the neighbourhood. Anastomoses connect all listed groups, and in this way, the extratrunkal veins are the vessels through which blood flows from the nerve trunk [1].

In Fig. 15.2, the extratrunkal part (1) of the vasa nervorum is present.

In Fig. 15.3, the epineural veins (1) after removal of the epineurium (2) are present. Veins are connected by many anastomoses. The largest of them (3) penetrates through the epineurium and opens into the extratrunkal veins. After removing the

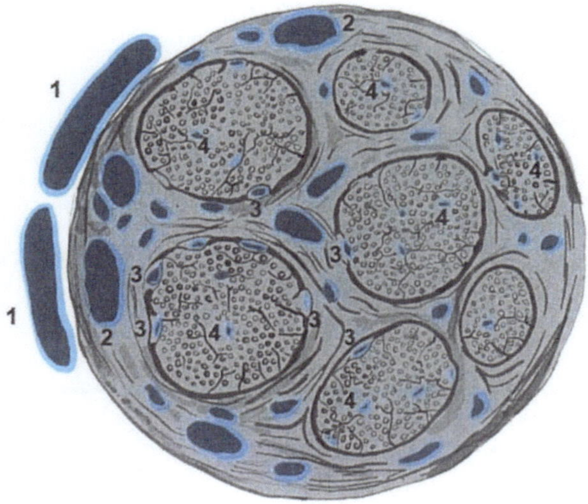

Fig. 15.1 Based on the topography, we distinguish between extratrunkal veins of nerve (1) and intratrunkal veins. The first occurs in the paraneural space and the second in the nerve sheaths (illustrated by Mrs. Anna Francová)

Z. Haviarová et al., *Peripheral Nervous System*,
https://doi.org/10.1007/978-3-031-73744-2_15

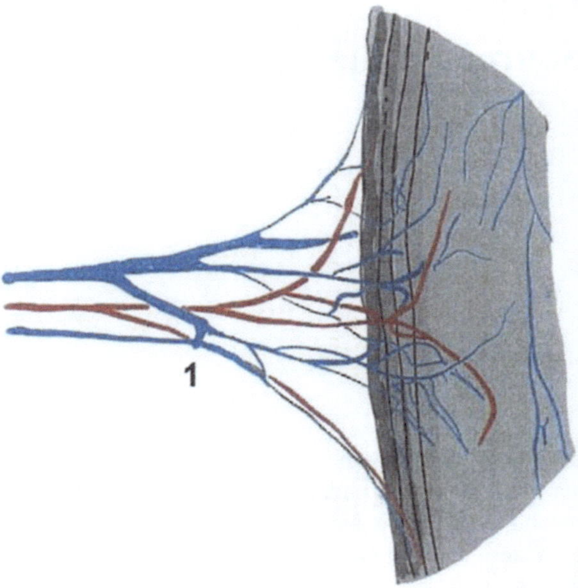

Fig. 15.2 Extratrunkal part (1) of nerve vessels (vasa nervorum) (illustrated by Ms. Anna Francová)

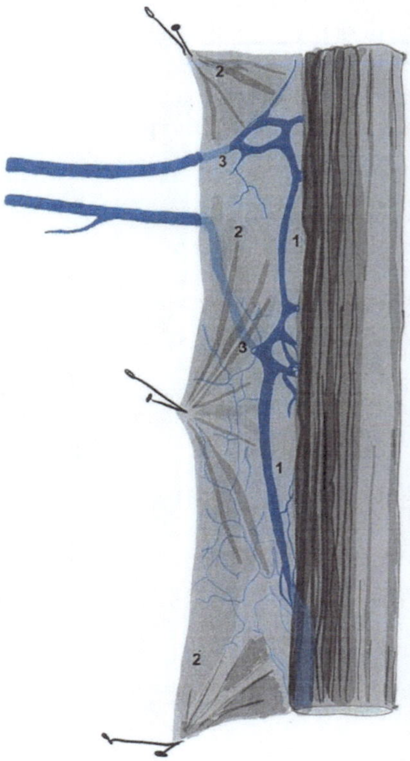

Fig. 15.3 Epineural veins (1) after removal of the epineurium (2). Veins are connected by many anastomoses. The largest of them (3) penetrates through the epineurium and opens into the extratrunkal veins (illustrated by Ms. Anna Francová)

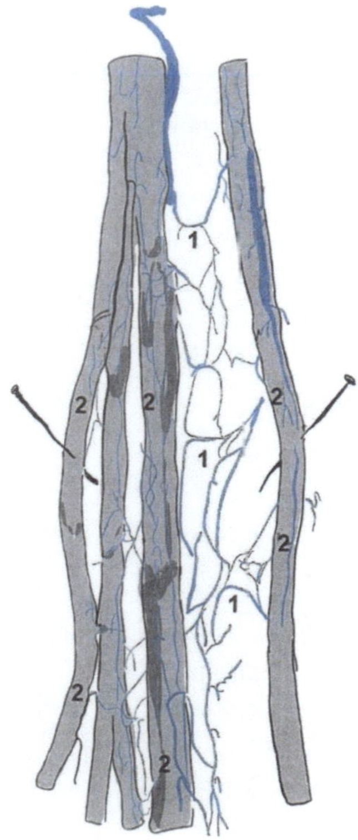

Fig. 15.4 After removing the epineurium of the nerve, multiple anastomoses can be seen between the epineural veins (1) and the perineural veins, from which epineural ones are formed (2) (illustrated by Ms. Anna Francová)

epineurium of the nerve, one can see (Fig. 15.4) multiple anastomoses between the epineural veins (1) and the perineural veins, which form the epineural veins (2). The presence of an extensive venous network surrounding the nerve and located in it also explains the changes observed in it during thrombosis, thrombophlebitis, and trauma.

Varicose changes also occur in the veins, both in the nerve itself and outside it. They appear with varicose veins on the limbs. In addition, varicose changes are observed in cases where the veins are collateral outflow pathways.

In several cases, we can observe varicose changes in the intratrunkal, especially the epineural vessels. In the case of varicose changes of the intratrunkal and extra-trunkal veins of the nerves in the nerve trunk itself, changes manifesting in their development and the development of connective elements and in the growth of the epineurium and the breakdown of myelin are observed.

Reference

1. Berthelot JM, Douane F, Ploteau S, Le Goff B, Darrieutort-Laffite C. Venous congestion as a central mechanism of radiculopathies. Joint Bone Spine. 2022;89(2):105291.

Chapter 16
Hematomas of Peripheral Nerves—Sources and Sequelae

Circumscribed, sometimes multiple hematomas are most often the result of traumatic rupture of thin-walled epineural veins [1]. In Fig. 16.1, several small circumscribed haemorrhages in the epineurium in the course of the epineural veins are seen.

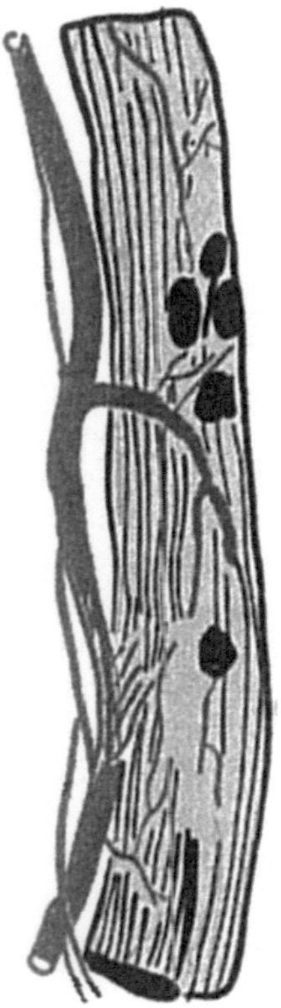

Fig. 16.1 Several small, circumscribed haemorrhages in the epineurium in the course of the epineural veins (illustrated by Ms. Anna Francová)

Z. Haviarová et al., *Peripheral Nervous System*,
https://doi.org/10.1007/978-3-031-73744-2_16

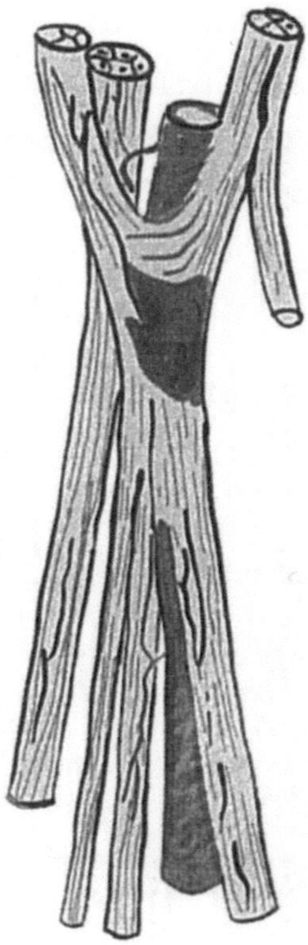

Fig. 16.2 Venous hematoma at the junction of the fascicles (illustrated by Ms. Anna Francová)

Similarly, one venous hematoma can be observed at the junction of the fascicles (Fig. 16.2).

In Fig. 16.3, there is another type of venous hematoma.

In the case of injuries near the nerve, the hematoma penetrates through all its coverings (blood imbibition) and has no clear borders. Such hematomas are the result of damage to both veins and arteries of the nerve.

In Figs. 16.4 and 16.5., another type of hematoma is seen.

In cases where the vein accompanying the nerve is damaged, the hematoma reaches large dimensions and can fill part or all spaces of the fascial sheath—the sleeve of the nerve (Figs. 16.6 and 16.7).

In the case of an extensive hematoma, a significant impairment of the motor and sensory functions of the nerve is observed. In superficial (epineural) hematomas, the disturbance of the motor and sensory functions of the nerve can be inconspicuous and tends to improve.

The expansion and pronounced tortuosity of the epineural veins near the nerve lesion can serve as an additional symptom of significant structural changes inside the nerve.

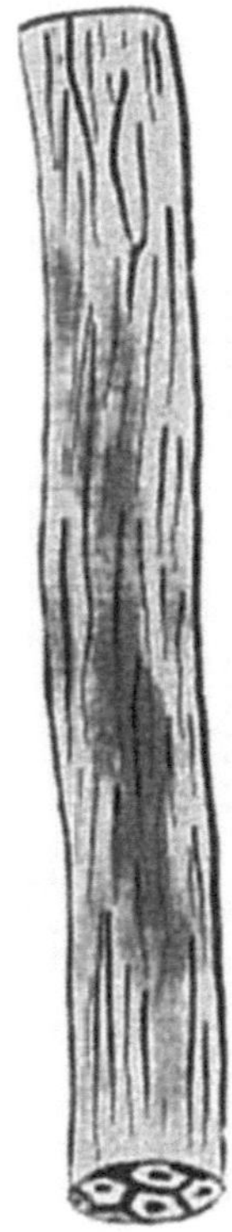

Fig. 16.3 Another type of venous hematoma (illustrated by Mrs. Anna Francová)

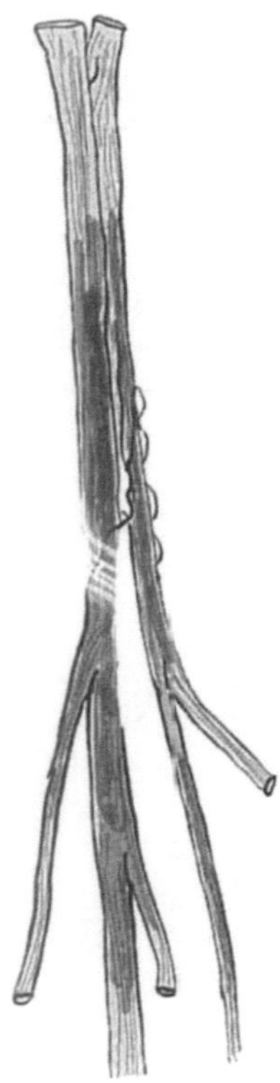

Fig. 16.4 Another type of hematoma (illustrated by Mrs. Anna Francová)

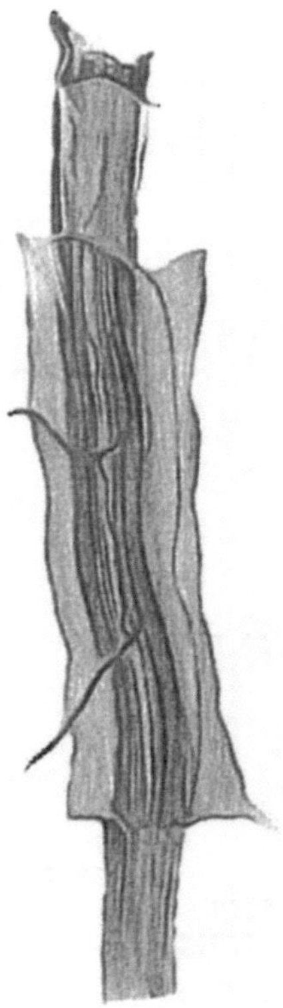

Fig. 16.5 Another type of hematoma (illustrated by Ms. Anna Francová)

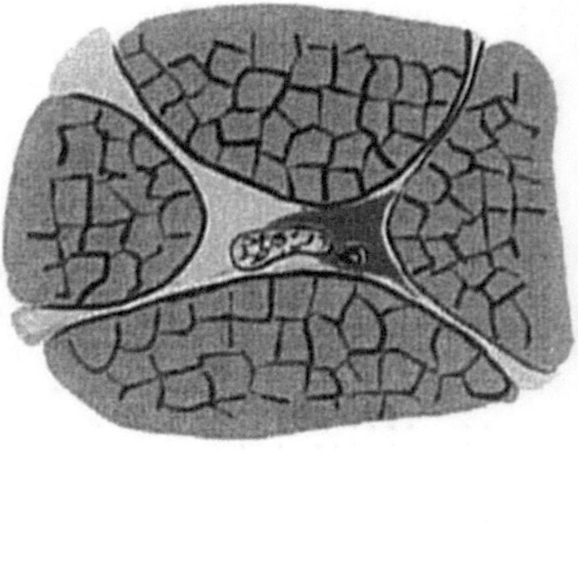

Fig. 16.6 Hematoma fills part of the space of the fascial sheath—nerve sheath (illustrated by Ms. Anna Francová)

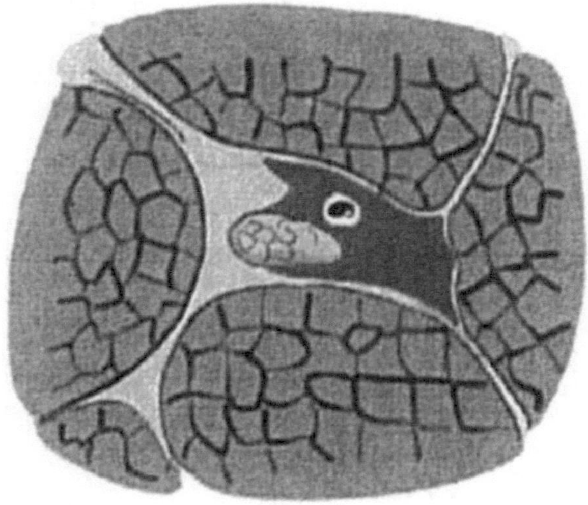

Fig. 16.7 Hematoma fills part of the space of the fascial sheath (illustrated by Ms. Anna Francová)

Reference

1. Berthelot JM, Douane F, Ploteau S, Le Goff B, Darrieutort-Laffite C. Venous congestion as a central mechanism of radiculopathies. Joint Bone Spine. 2022;89(2):105291.

Part VI
Conclusion

Chapter 17
Summary of Our Contribution

This monograph is one of the few documents that comprehensively evaluate the topic of morphological and clinical aspects of the entire peripheral nervous system. It provides information on its topography, morphology, and especially features that are missing in anatomical textbooks [1, 2]. We did not find any detailed studies regarding the description of variations—peculiarities of the whole peripheral nervous system.

Surgical practice requires the knowledge of anatomical structures, their location, and topographical relationships. Pictures and line drawings enrich the view of structures that have only been partially documented so far, even though some are difficult to visualize due to their small dimensions. Dissection provides an important three-dimensional view, elucidating the range of variability and demonstrating interdisciplinary connections and relationships between the anatomy and surgical disciplines.

In our work, we evaluate the peculiarities of the peripheral nervous system, including the cranial autonomic ganglia, and their significance for surgical disciplines. We are interested in ensuring that the potential of the acquired knowledge does not remain unused and does not lead to the isolation of preclinical disciplines such as anatomy. We believe that our work will contribute to a better understanding of the topic and that the data obtained will be helpful not only to surgeons.

The results of anatomical variation studies are important for a more accurate interpretation of perioperative and clinical findings and are the means to achieve the goal of perfect patient treatment. Our observations, which we present in this book, are the result of clinical observations and systematic work on the cadavers of previously healthy people who died suddenly or violently (most often in car accidents).

The work on the variations of the peripheral autonomic system allowed us to describe anatomical variations that clarify often unexpected clinical findings during clinical examinations. This work follows from our previous works on variations in the peripheral nervous system.

Z. Haviarová et al., *Peripheral Nervous System*,
https://doi.org/10.1007/978-3-031-73744-2_17

The work aimed to bring closer the morphological and clinical aspects of the peculiarities of the peripheral nervous system and its peculiarities not only from the anatomical diagnostic and differential diagnostic but also from the clinical point of view. We hope that this book has fulfilled its purpose and that it can become a useful text for deepening the knowledge of students and doctors or for compiling further professional literature on the mentioned issue. We believe that we have managed to sufficiently describe the various symptoms and manifestations of the disease, and the publication will be of benefit to the reader in the study of the given complicated issue.

References

1. Lovásová K, Šulla IJ, Boleková A, Šulla I, Kluchová D. Anatomical study of the roots of cranial parasympathetic ganglia: a contribution to medical education. Ann Anat. 2013;195(3):205–11.
2. Shiozawa T, Herlan S, Wagner HJ, Küppers E. Surgical prosection in a traditional anatomical curriculum-Tübingens' Sectio chirurgica. Ann Anat. 2010;192(6):349–54.

Chapter 18
Supplementary Figures

Lesions of the Peripheral Nerves of the Upper Limbs

See Figs. 18.1, 18.2, 18.3, 18.4, 18.5, 18.6, 18.7, 18.8, 18.9, 18.10, 18.11, 18.12, 18.13, 18.14, 18.15, 18.16, 18.17, 18.18, 18.19 and 18.20.

Z. Haviarová et al., *Peripheral Nervous System*,
https://doi.org/10.1007/978-3-031-73744-2_18

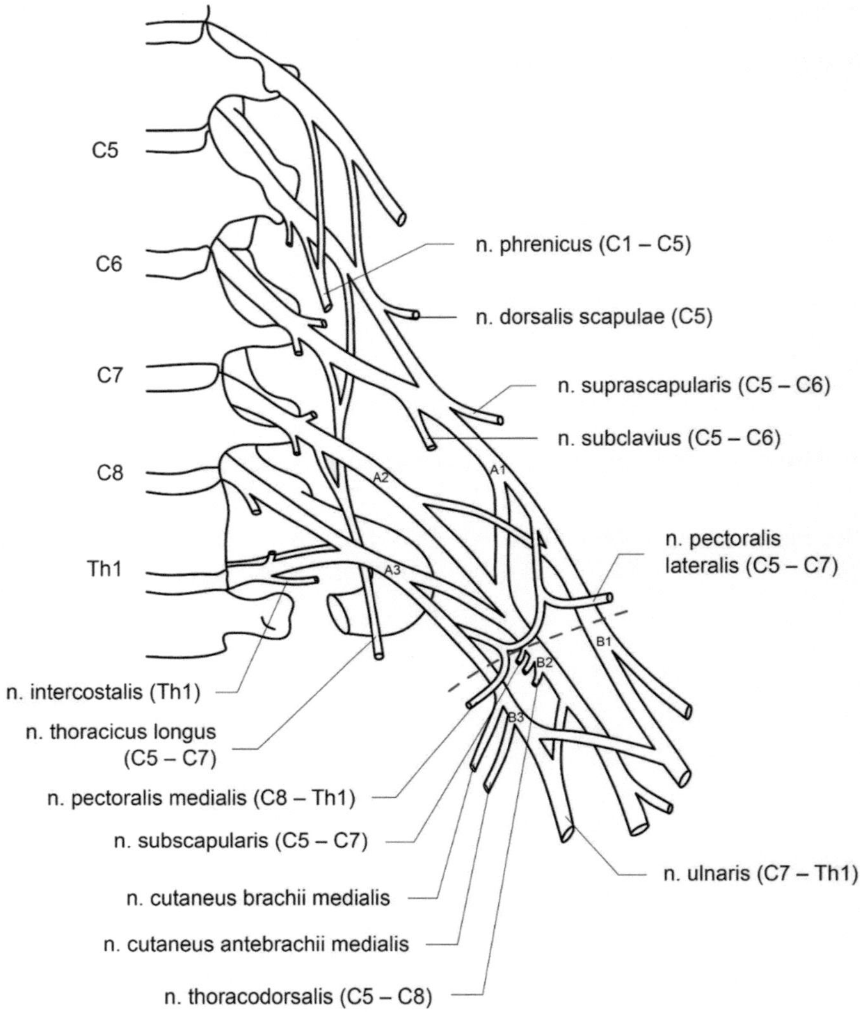

Fig. 18.1 Brachial plexus—formation (illustrated by Ms. Anna Francová)

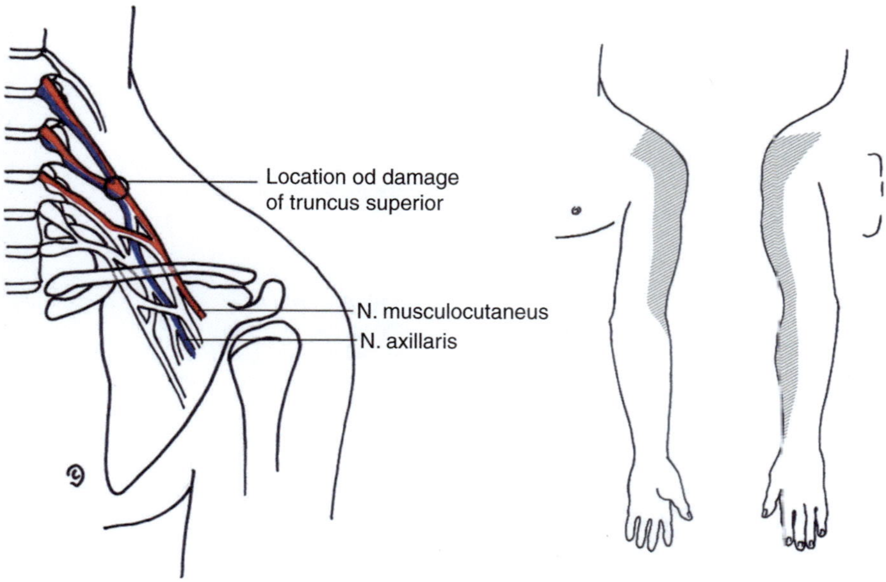

Fig. 18.2 Superior trunk lesion—clinical symptoms (illustrated by Ms. Anna Francová)

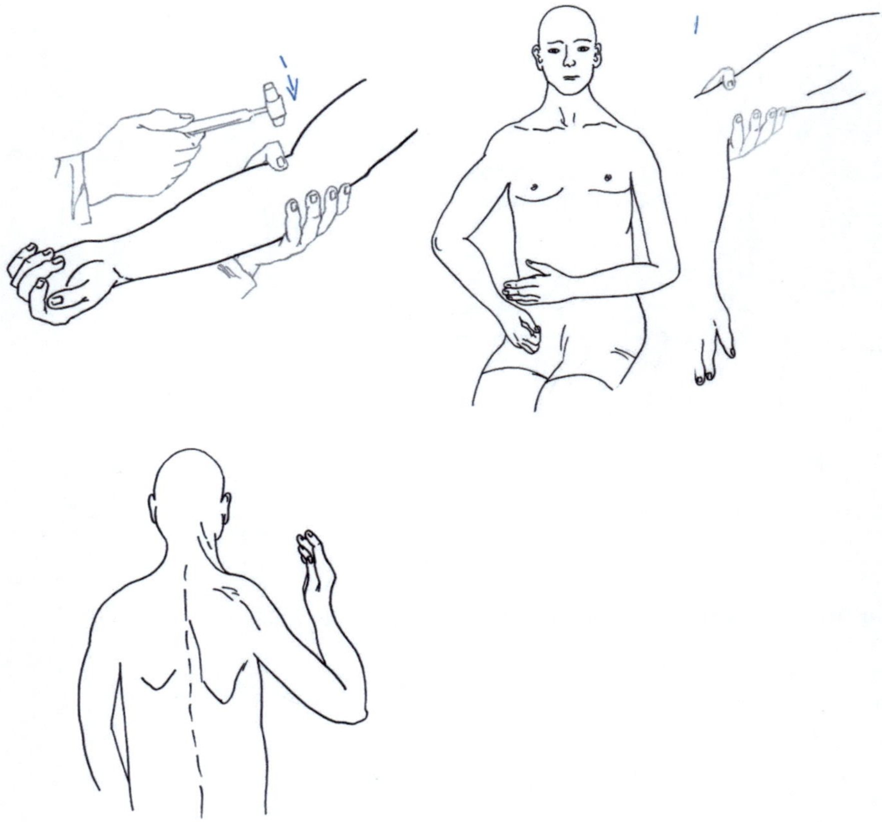

Fig. 18.3 Superior trunk lesion—clinical symptoms (illustrated by Ms. Anna Francová)

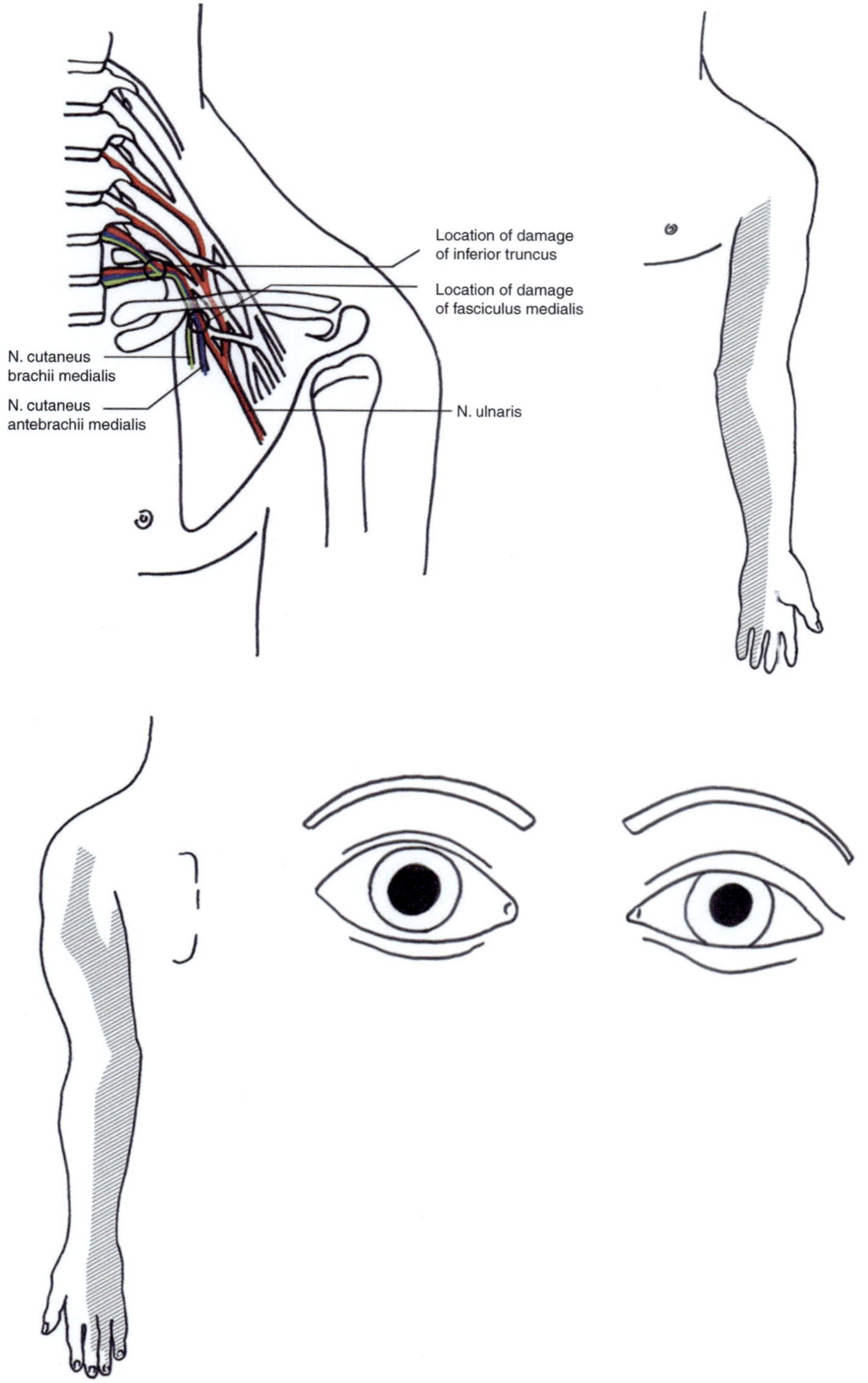

Fig. 18.4 Lesion of the inferior trunk and medial fascicle (fasciculus medialis)—clinical symptoms (illustrated by Ms. Anna Francová)

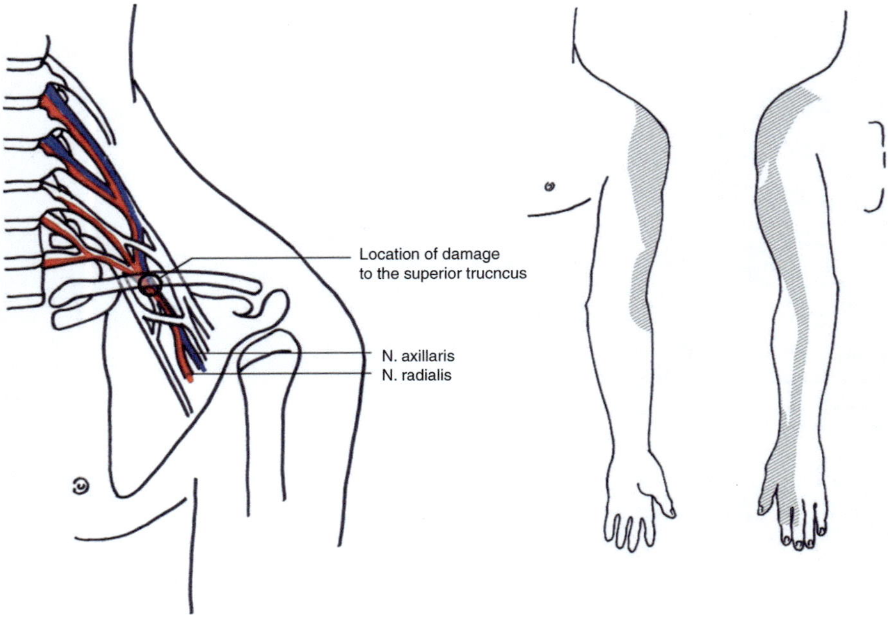

Fig. 18.5 Posterior fascicle lesion—clinical symptoms (illustrated by Ms. Anna Francová)

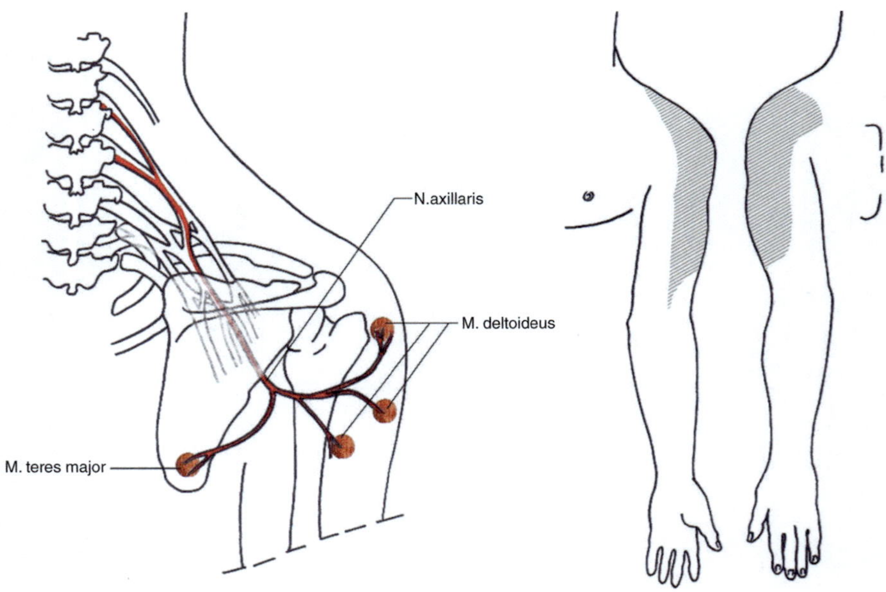

Fig. 18.6 Posterior fascicle lesion—clinical symptoms (illustrated by Ms. Anna Francová)

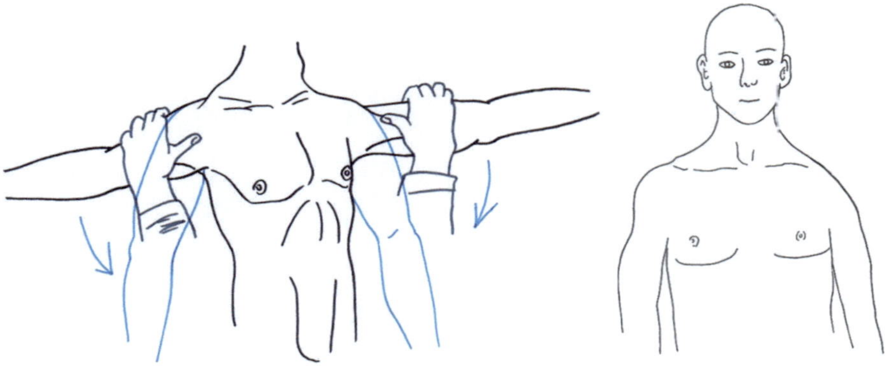

Fig. 18.7 Lesion of the axillary nerve—clinical symptoms (illustrated by Ms. Anna Francová)

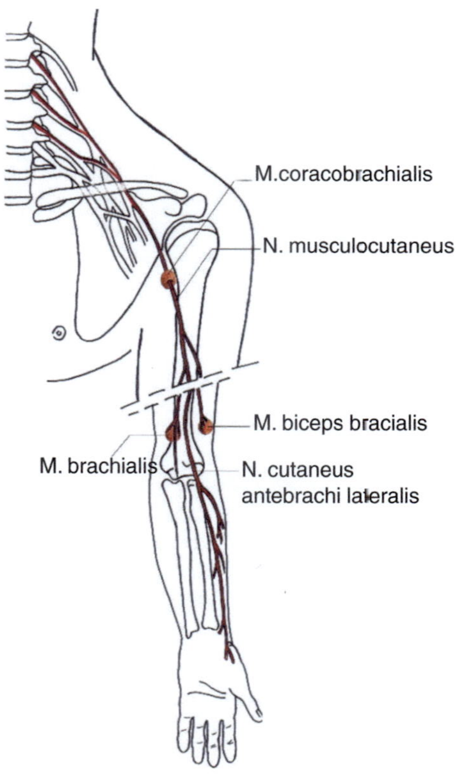

Fig. 18.8 Lesion of musculocutaneus nerve—innervation area (illustrated by Ms. Anna Francová)

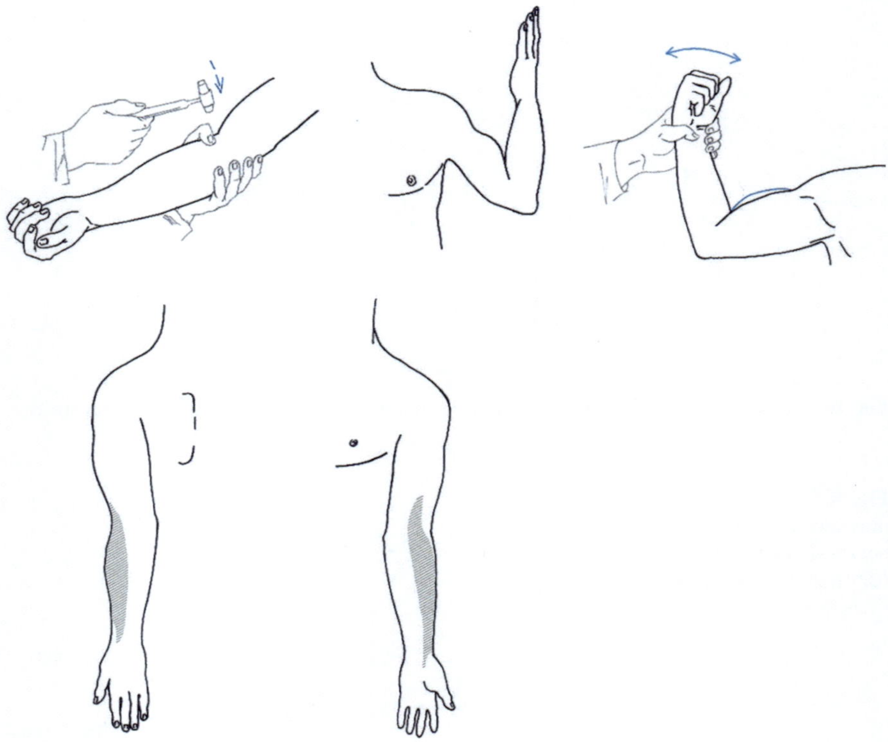

Fig. 18.9 Lesion of the musculocutaneus nerve—clinical symptoms (illustrated by Ms. Anna Francová)

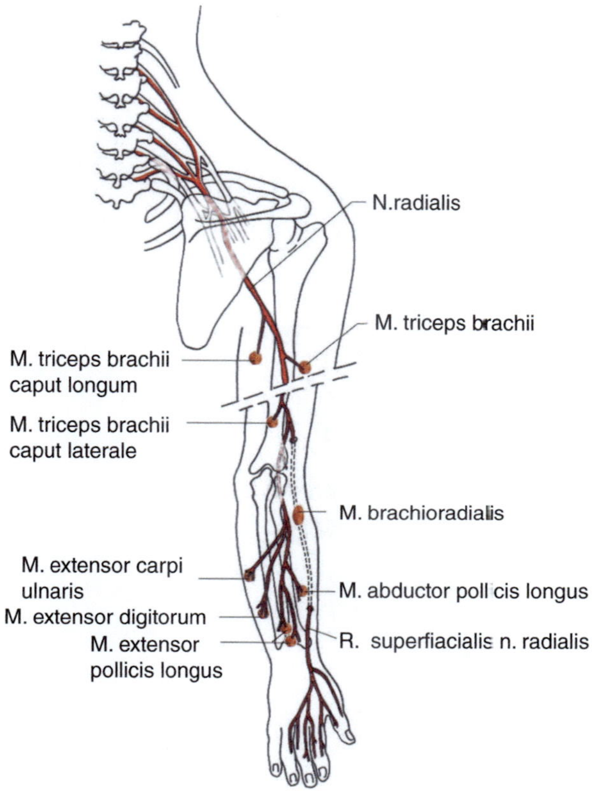

Fig. 18.10 Lesion of radial nerve—innervation area (illustrated by Ms. Anna Francová)

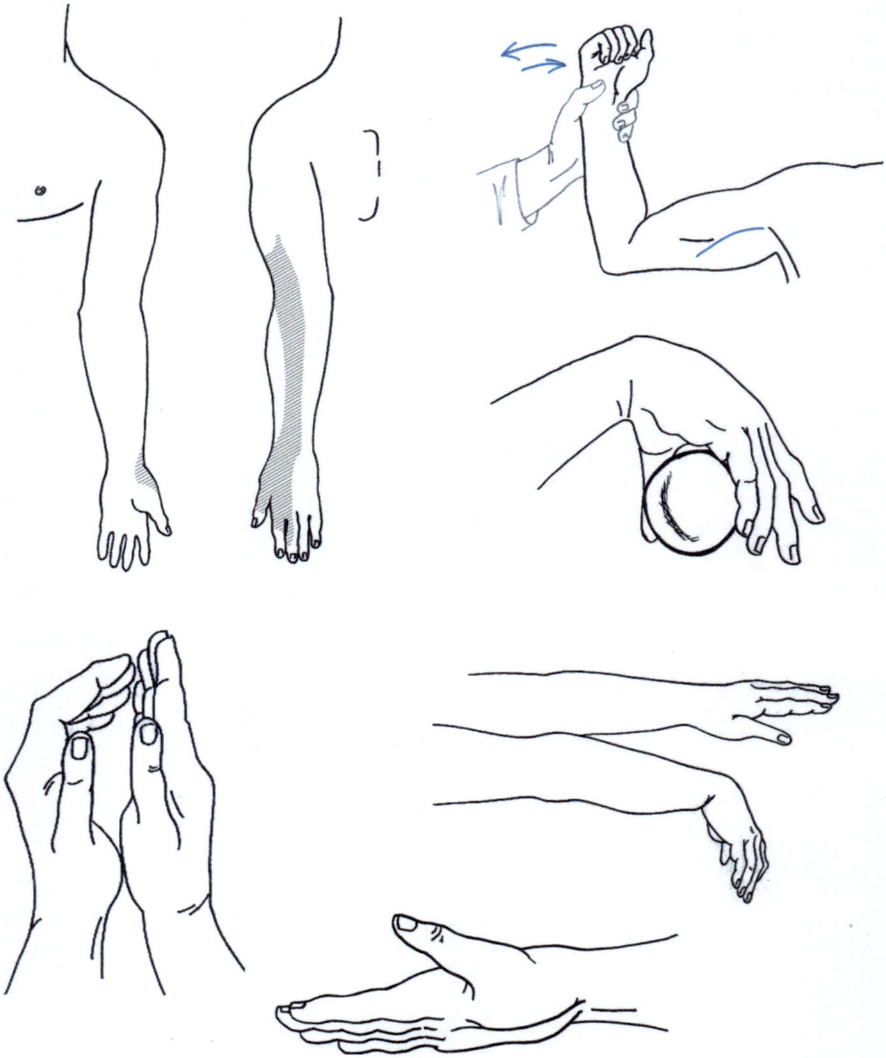

Fig. 18.11 Lesion of radial nerve—clinical symptoms (illustrated by Ms. Anna Francová)

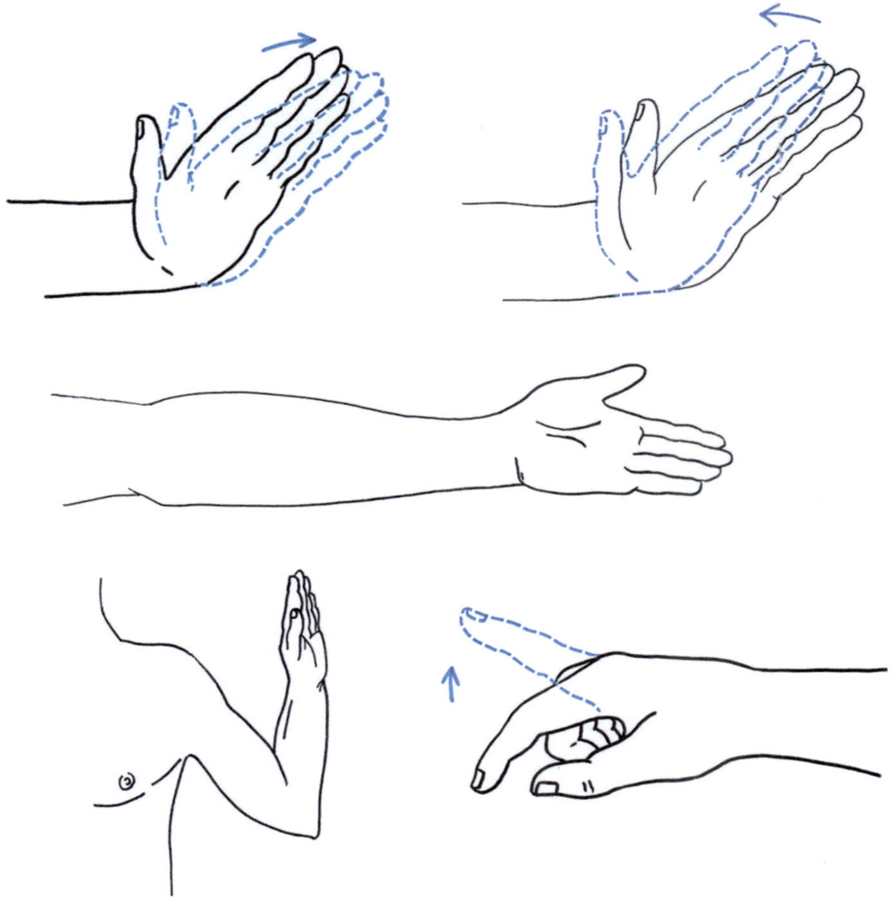

Fig. 18.12 Lesion of radial nerve—clinical symptoms (illustrated by Ms. Anna Francová)

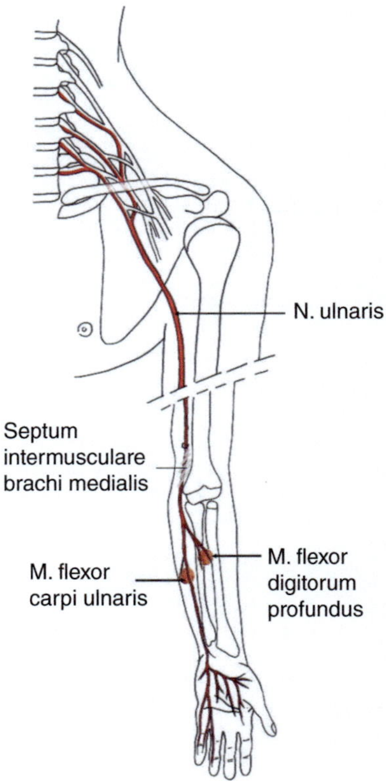

Fig. 18.13 Lesion of ulnar nerve—innervation area (illustrated by Ms. Anna Francová)

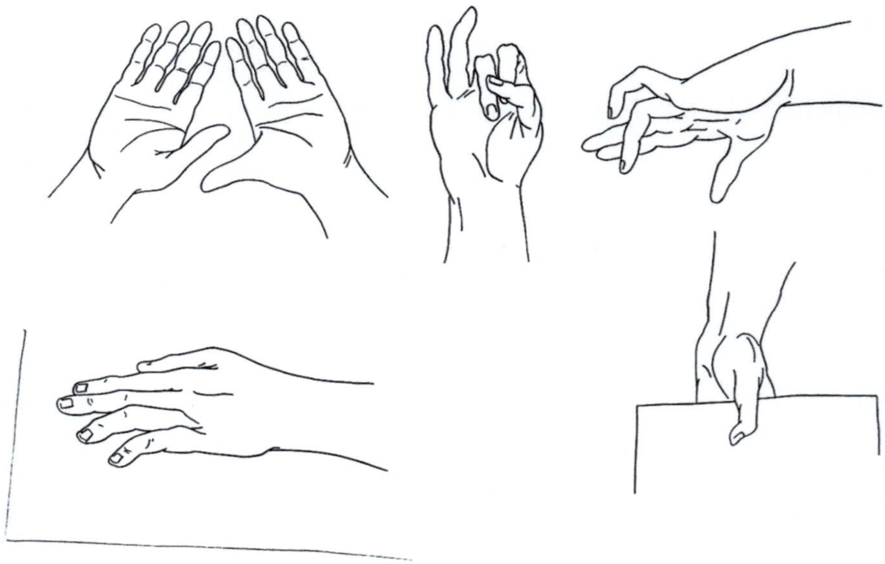

Fig. 18.14 Lesion of the ulnar nerve—clinical symptoms (illustrated by Ms. Anna Francová)

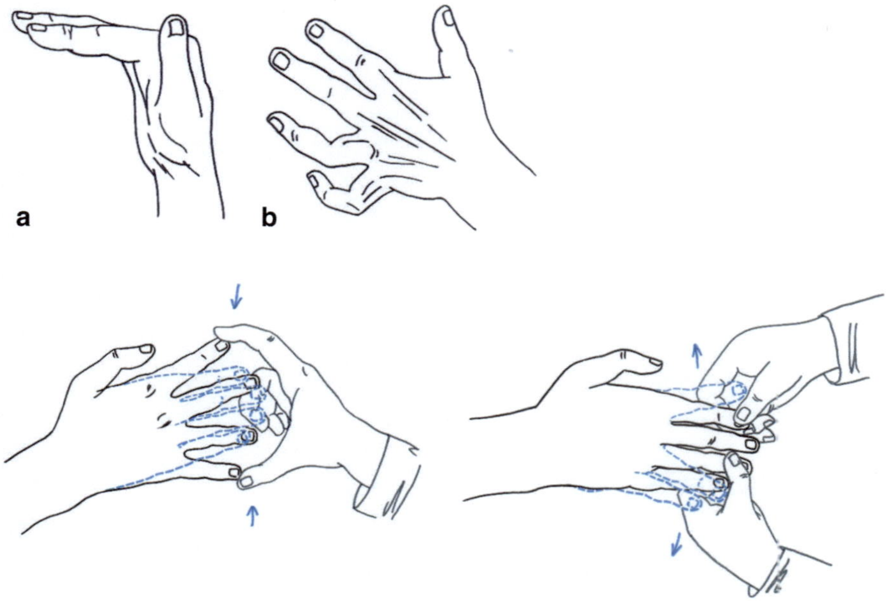

Fig. 18.15 Lesion of the ulnar nerve—clinical symptoms (illustrated by Ms. Anna Francová)

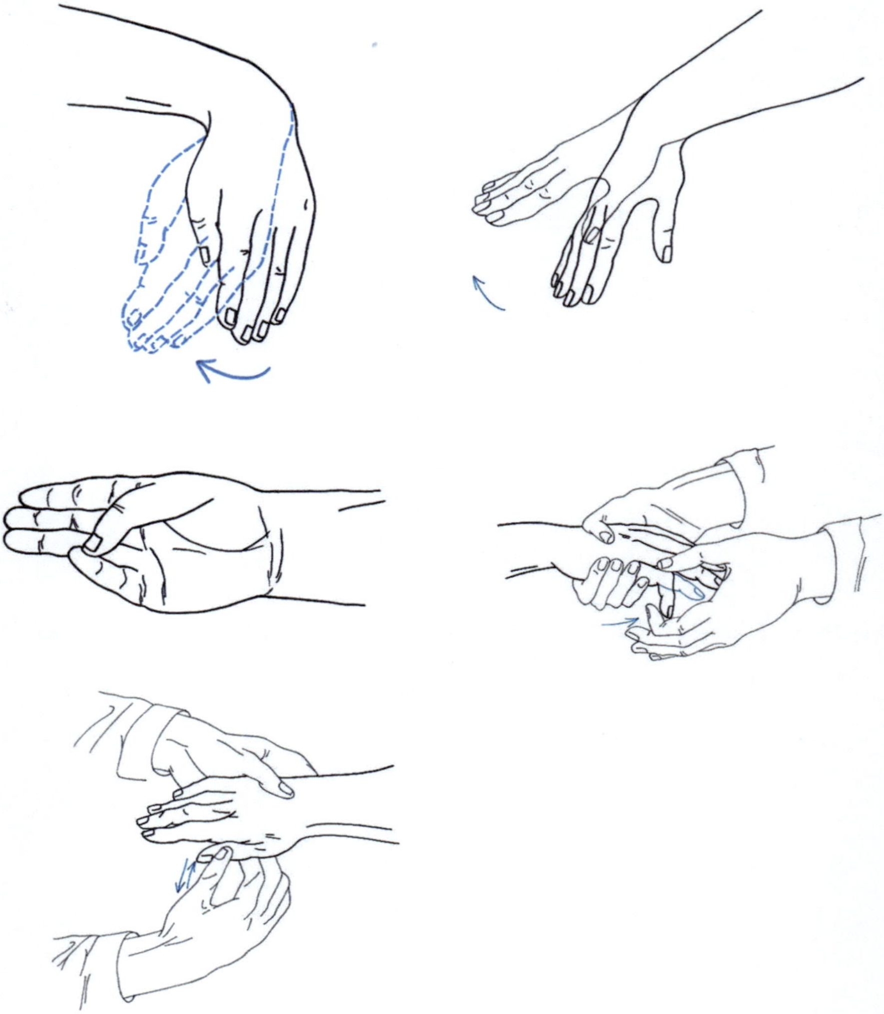

Fig. 18.16 Lesion of the ulnar nerve—clinical symptoms (illustrated by Ms. Anna Francová)

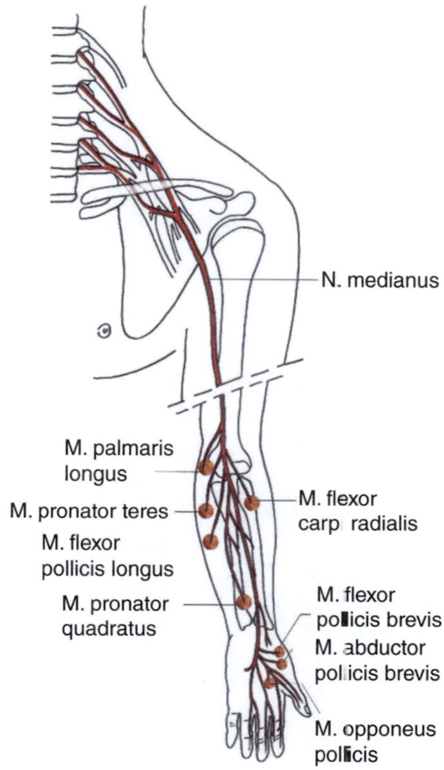

Fig. 18.17 Lesion of median nerve—innervation area (illustrated by Ms. Anna Francová)

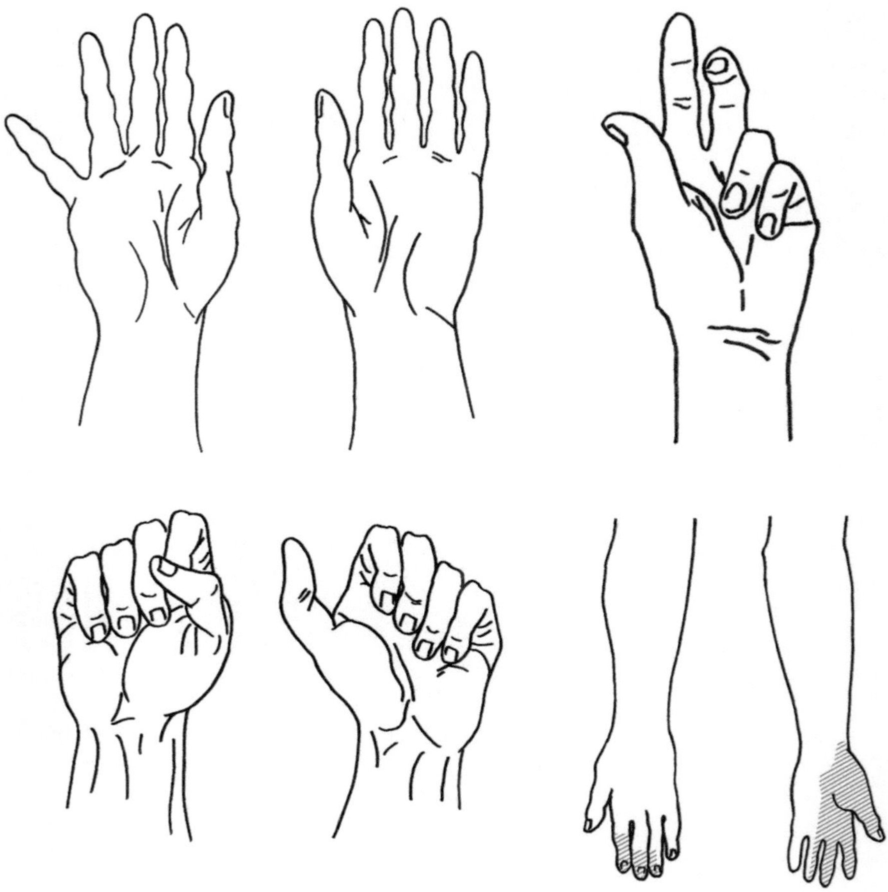

Fig. 18.18 Lesion of the median nerve—clinical symptoms (illustrated by Ms. Anna Francová)

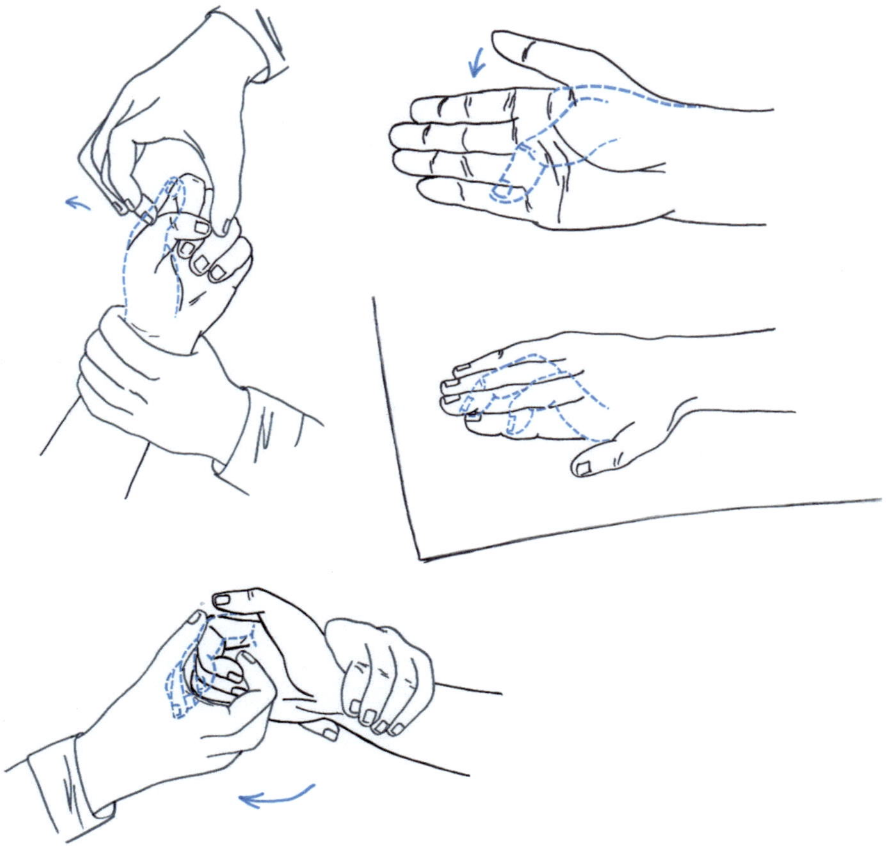

Fig. 18.19 Lesion of median nerve—clinical symptoms (illustrated by Ms. Anna Francová)

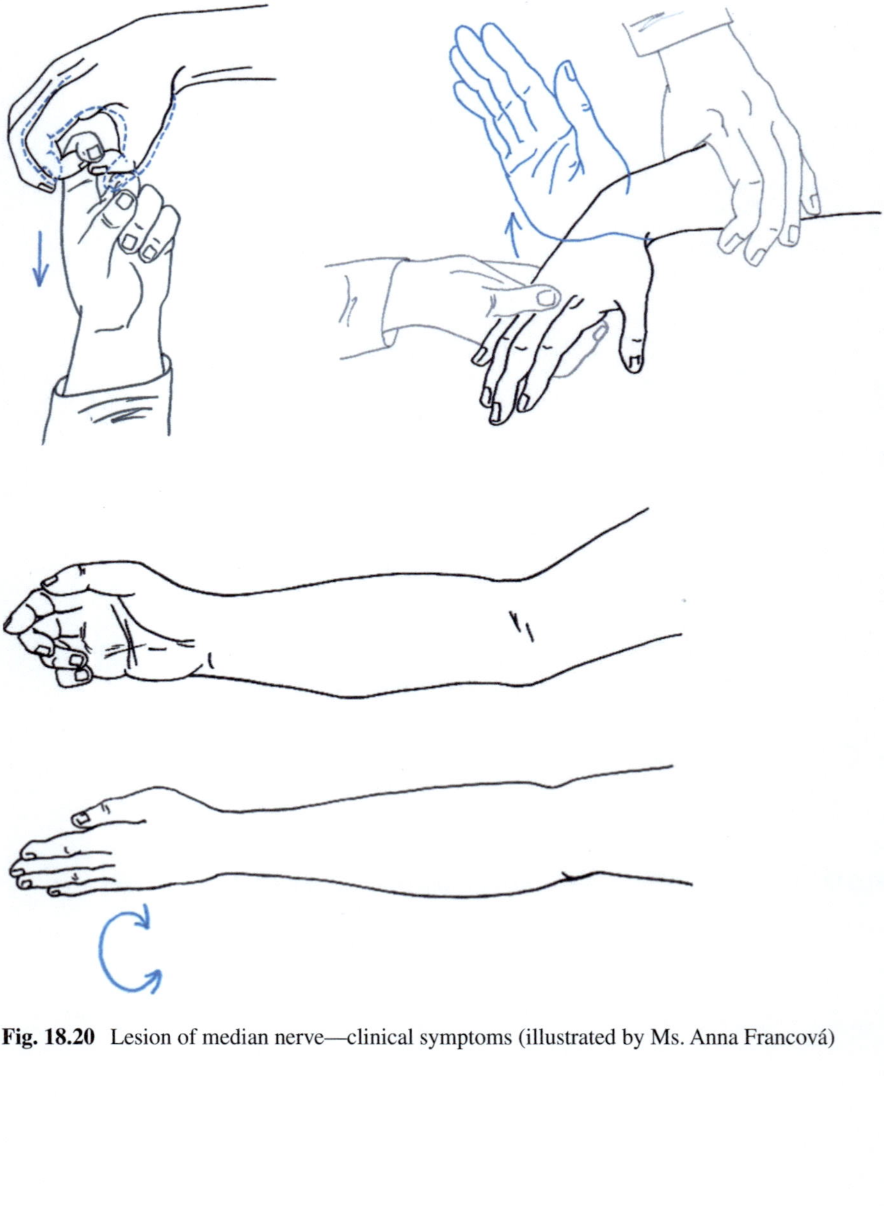

Fig. 18.20 Lesion of median nerve—clinical symptoms (illustrated by Ms. Anna Francová)

Lesions of the Peripheral Nerves of the Lower Limbs

See Figs. 18.21, 18.22, 18.23, 18.24, 18.25, 18.26, 18.27, 18.28, 18.29, 18.30, 18.31, 18.32, 18.33, 18.34, 18.35, 18.36, 18.37, 18.38, 18.39, 18.40, 18.41, 18.42, 18.43, 18.44, 18.45, 18.46, 18.47, 18.48, 18.49.

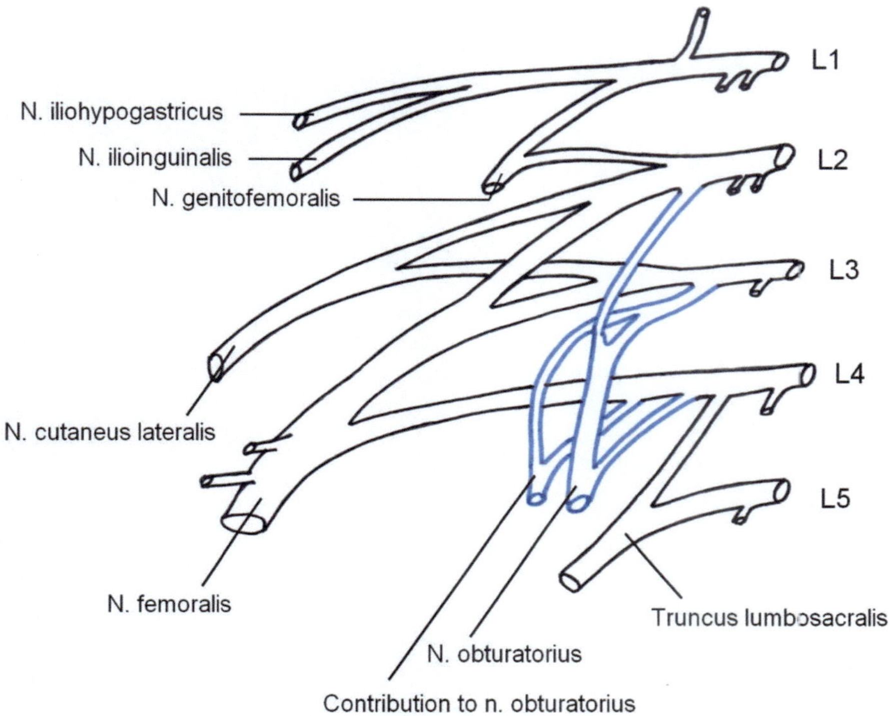

Fig. 18.21 Lumbar plexus (illustrated by Ms. Anna Francová)

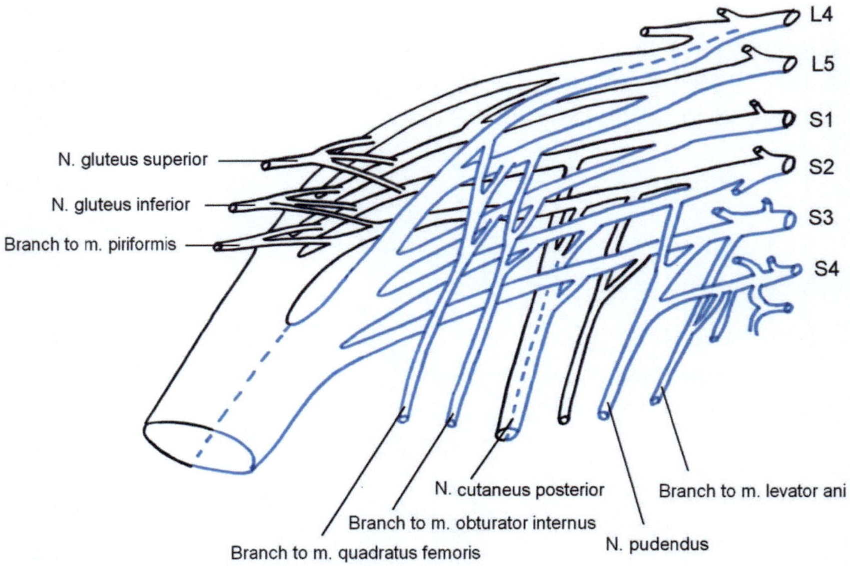

Fig. 18.22 Sacral plexus (illustrated by Ms. Anna Francová)

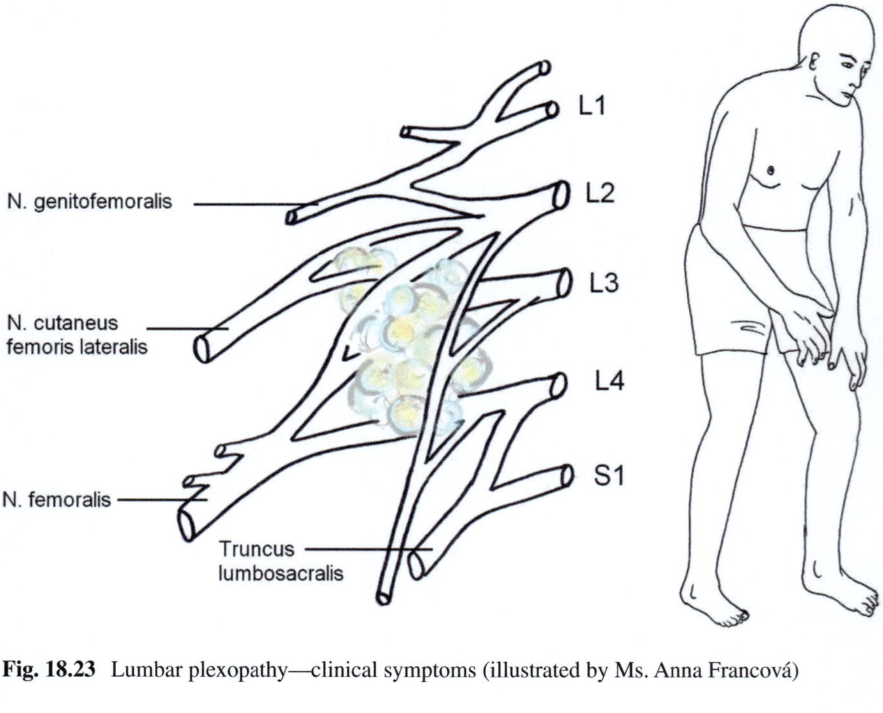

Fig. 18.23 Lumbar plexopathy—clinical symptoms (illustrated by Ms. Anna Francová)

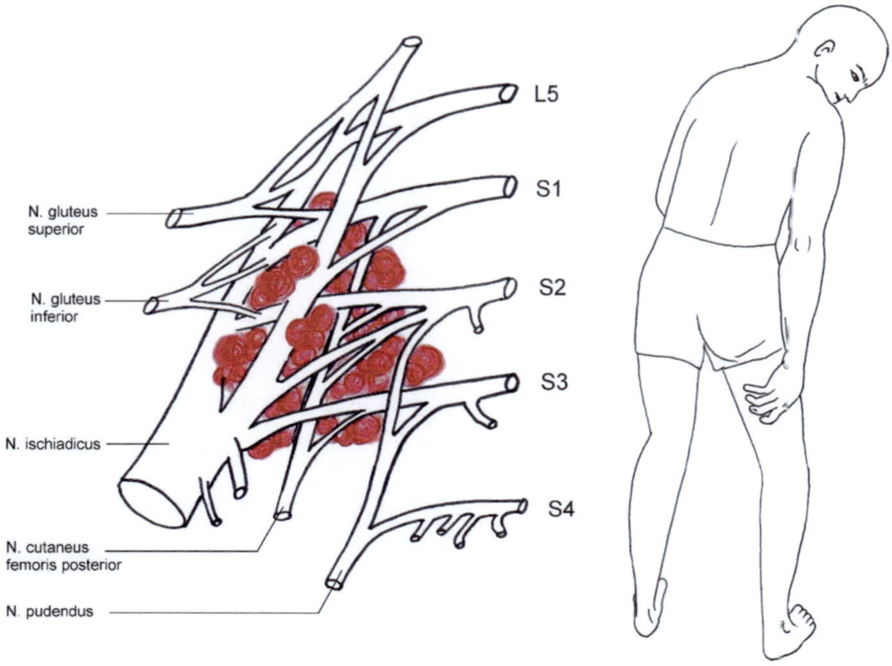

Fig. 18.24 Sacral plexopathy—clinical symptoms (illustrated by Ms. Anna Francová)

Fig. 18.25 Lesion of the sciatic nerve—clinical symptoms (illustrated by Ms. Anna Francová)

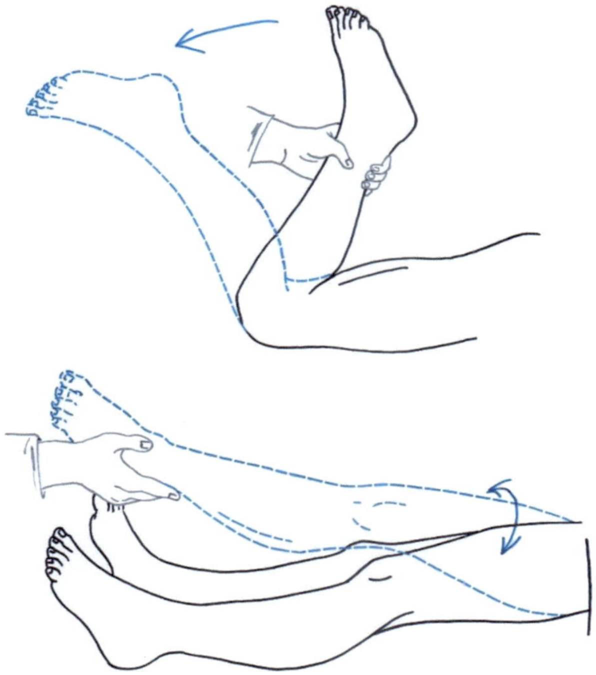

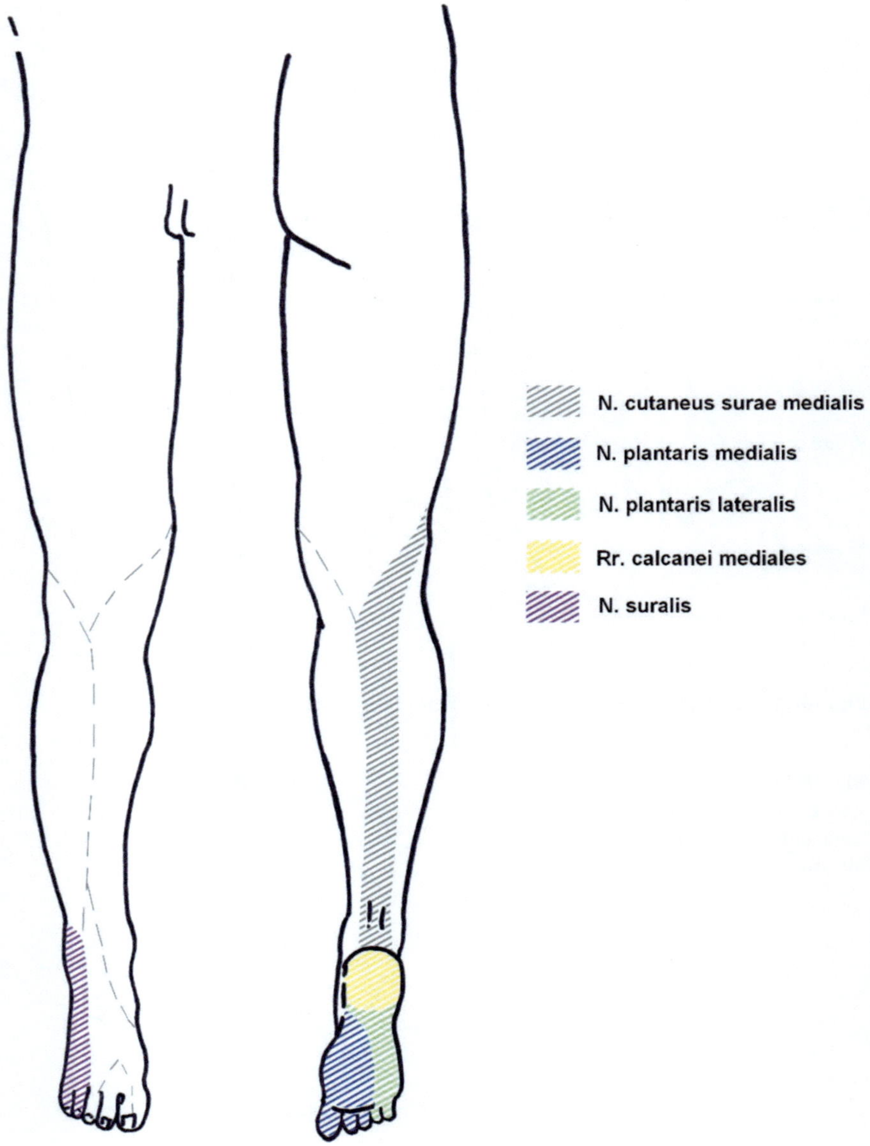

Fig. 18.26 Lesion of the sciatic nerve—clinical symptoms, areas of sensitivity disorders (illustrated by Ms. Anna Francová)

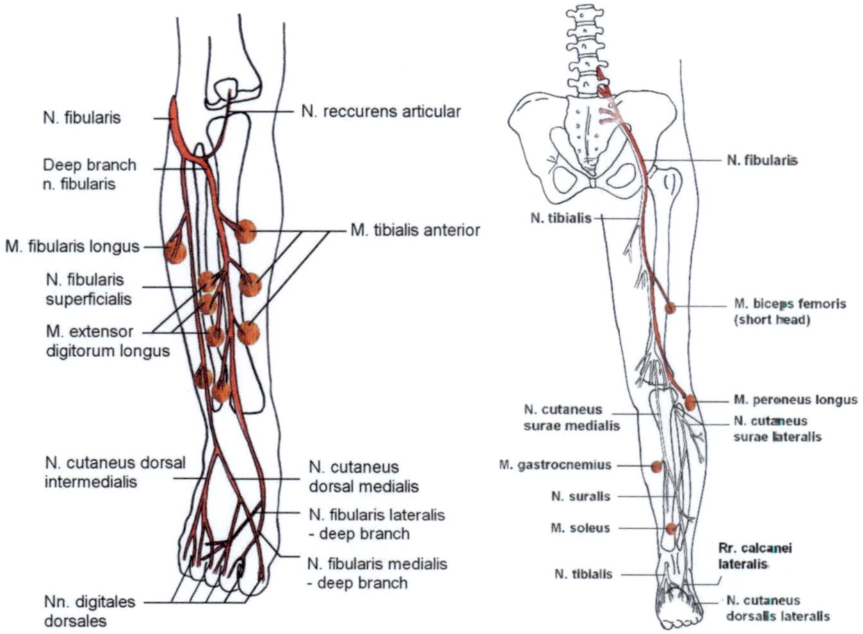

Fig. 18.27 Lesion of the sciatic nerve—innervation area (illustrated by Ms. Anna Francová)

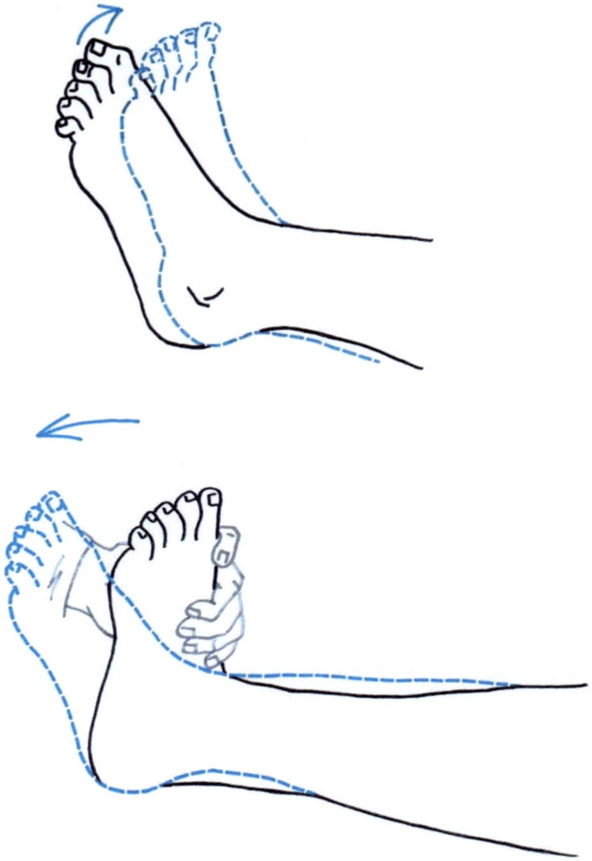

Fig. 18.28 Lesion of the fibular nerve—clinical symptoms (illustrated by Ms. Anna Francová)

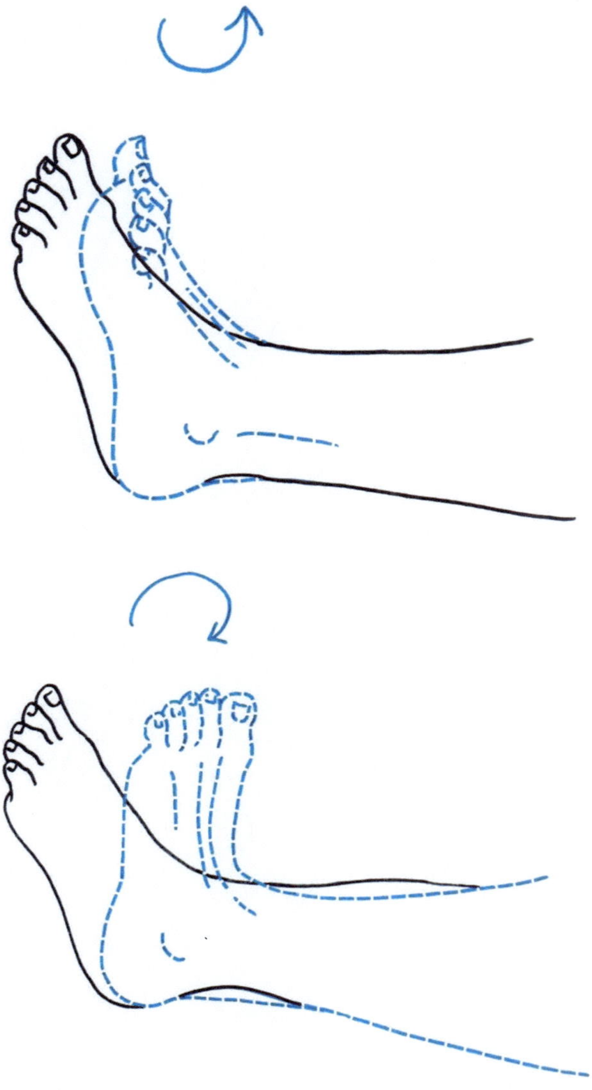

Fig. 18.28 (continued)

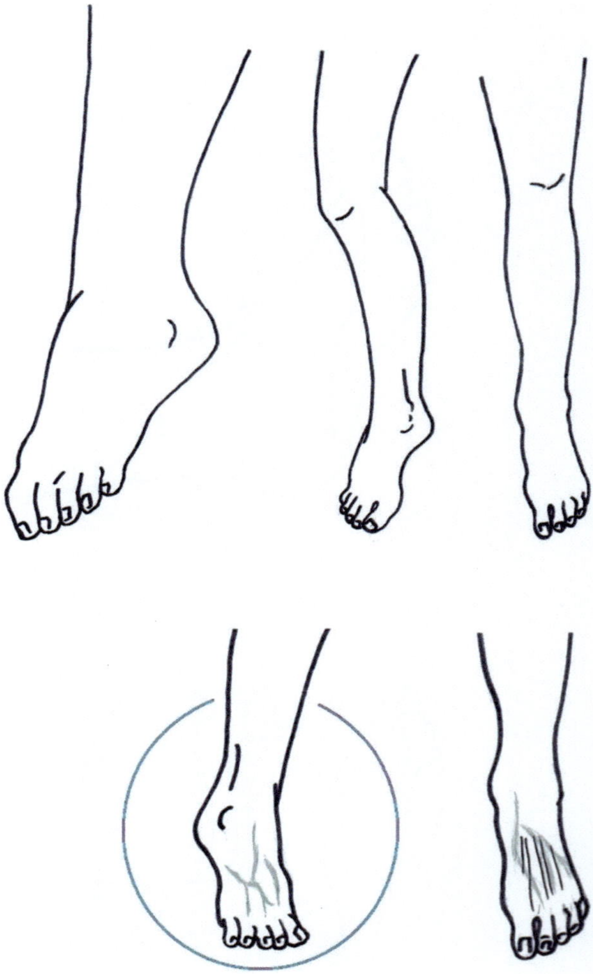

Fig. 18.29 Lesion of the fibular nerve—clinical symptoms (illustrated by Ms. Anna Francová)

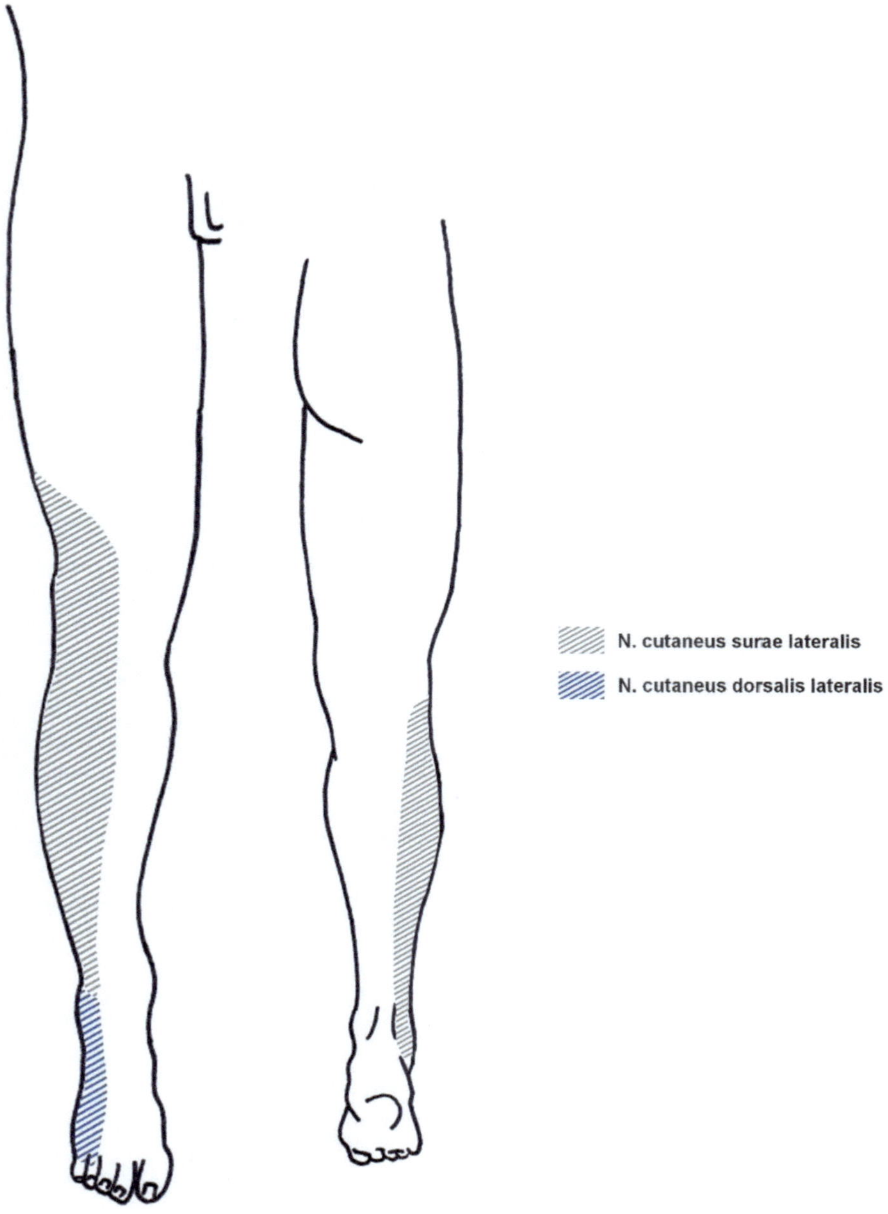

Fig. 18.30 Lesion of the fibular nerve—clinical symptoms (illustrated by Ms. Anna Francová)

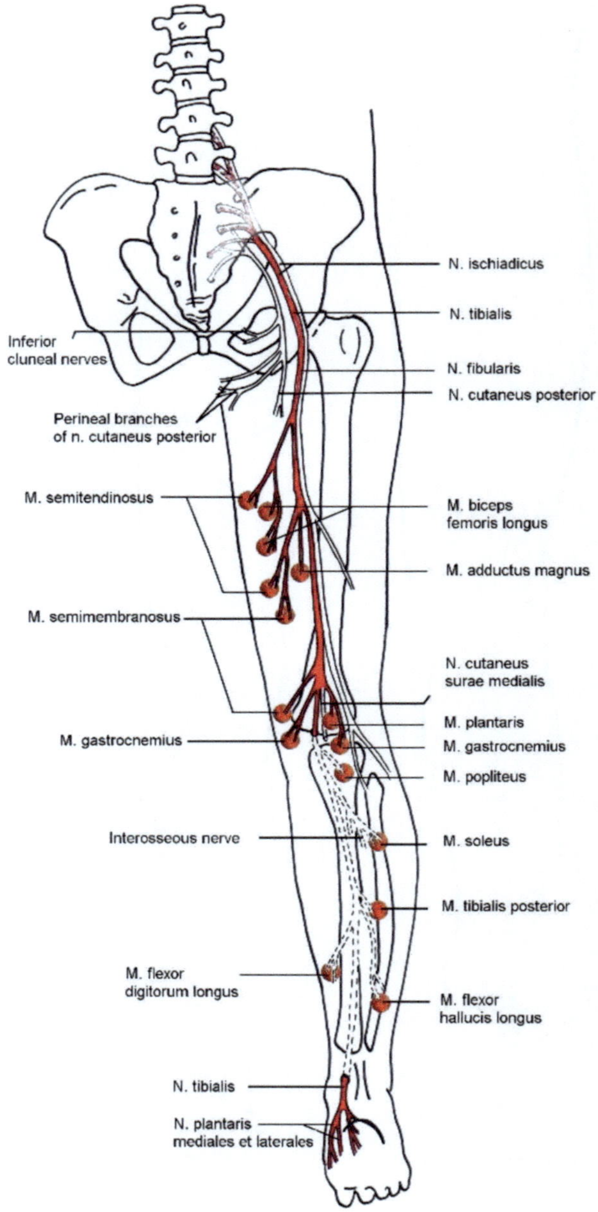

Fig. 18.31 Lesion of tibial nerve—innervation area (illustrated by Ms. Anna Francová)

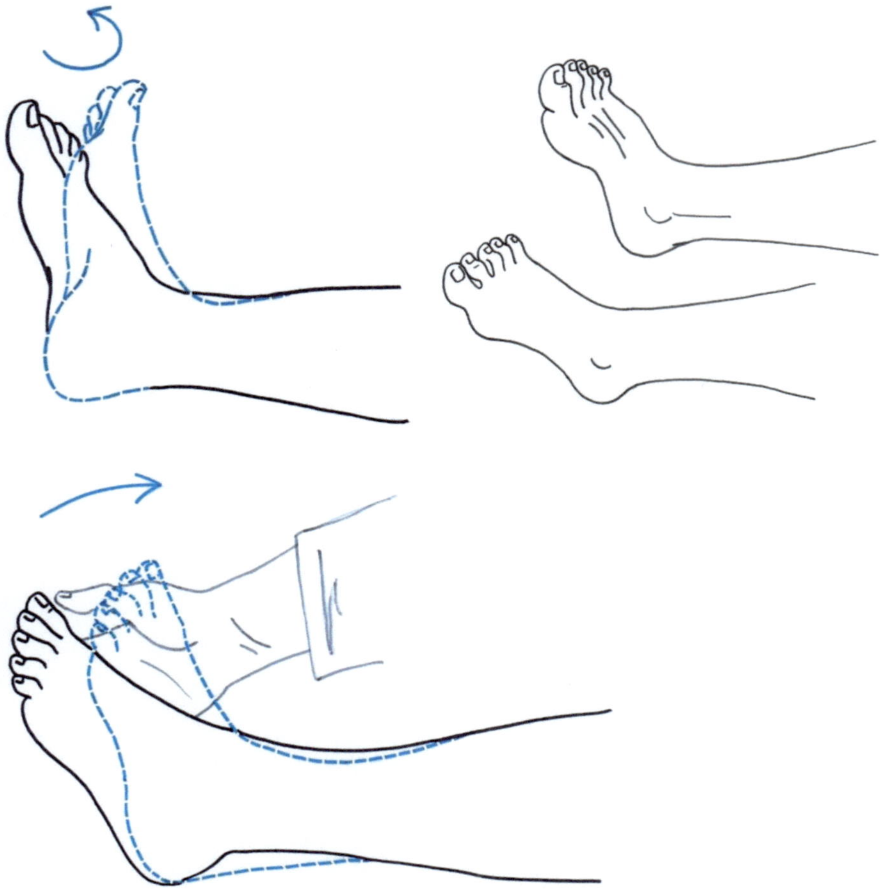

Fig. 18.32 Lesion of the tibial nerve—clinical symptoms (illustrated by Ms. Anna Francová)

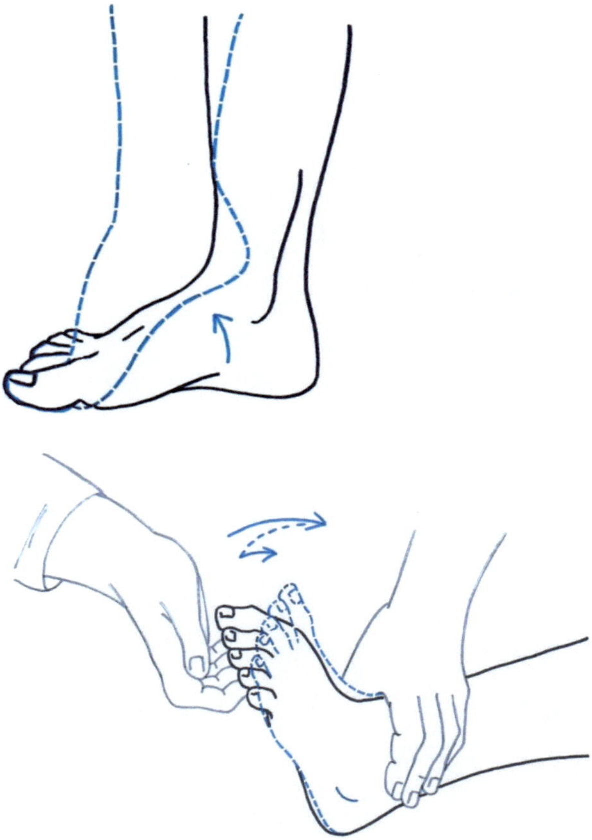

Fig. 18.32 (continued)

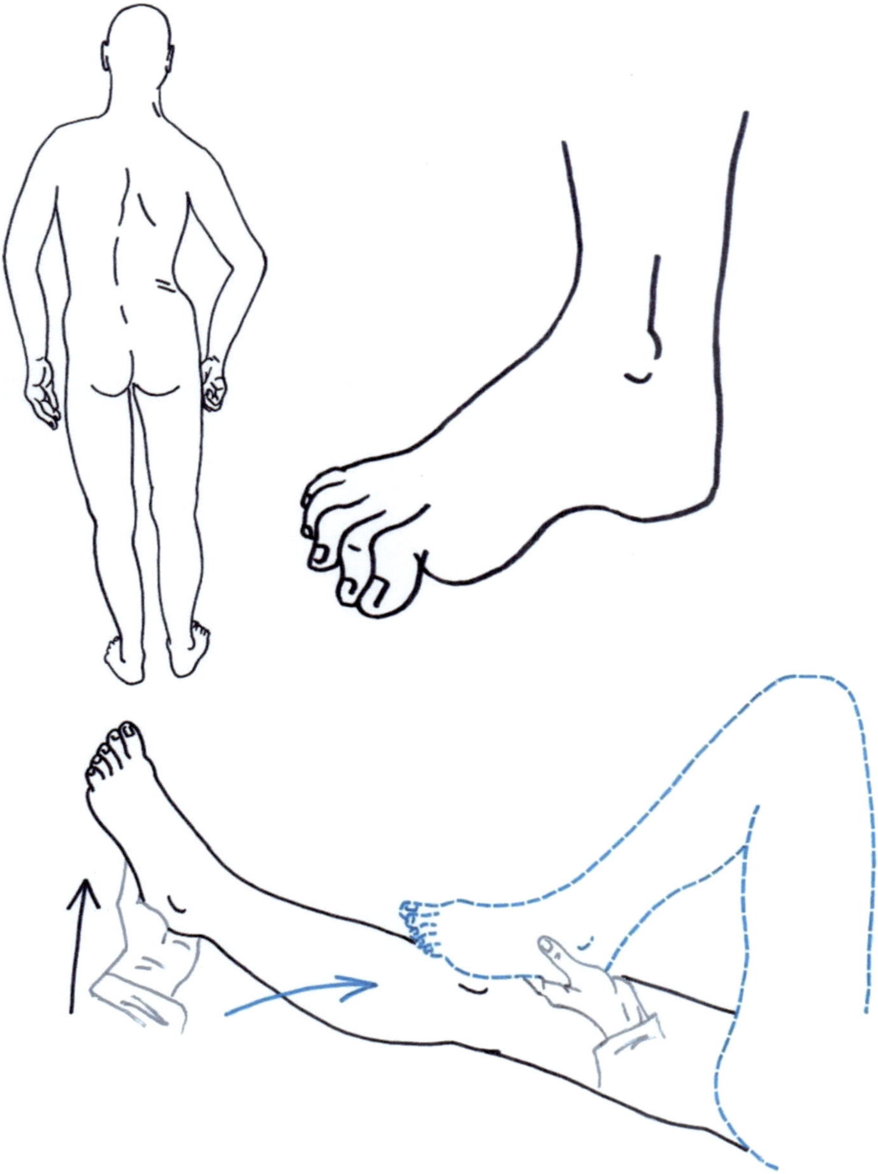

Fig. 18.33 Lesion of the tibial nerve—clinical symptoms (illustrated by Ms. Anna Francová)

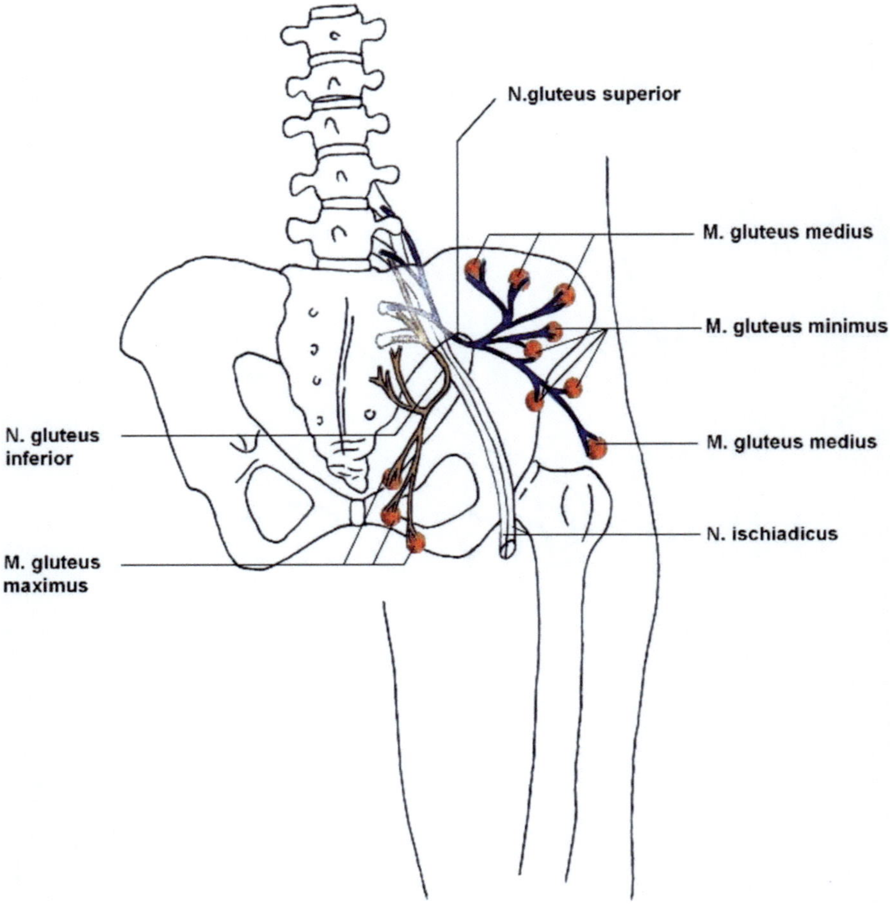

Fig. 18.34 Superior and inferior gluteal nerves—innervation areas (illustrated by Mrs. Anna Francová)

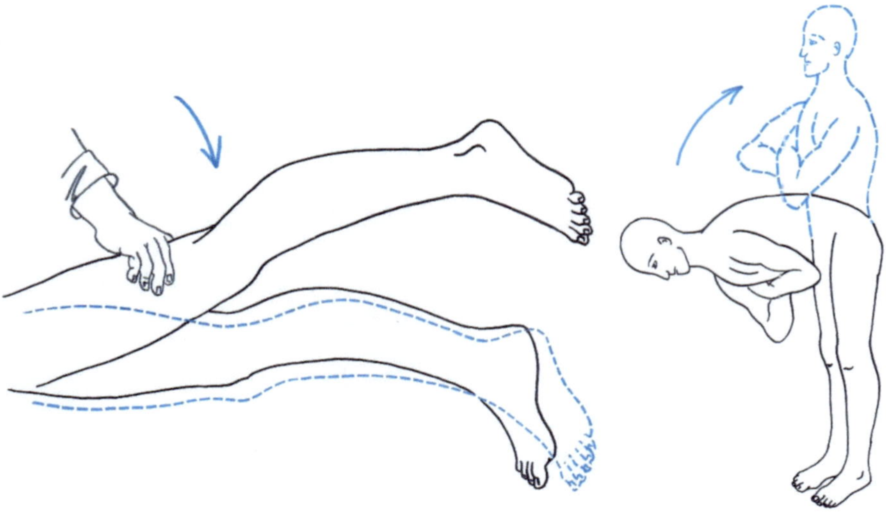

Fig. 18.35 Lesion of the inferior gluteal nerve—clinical symptoms (illustrated by Ms. Anna Francová)

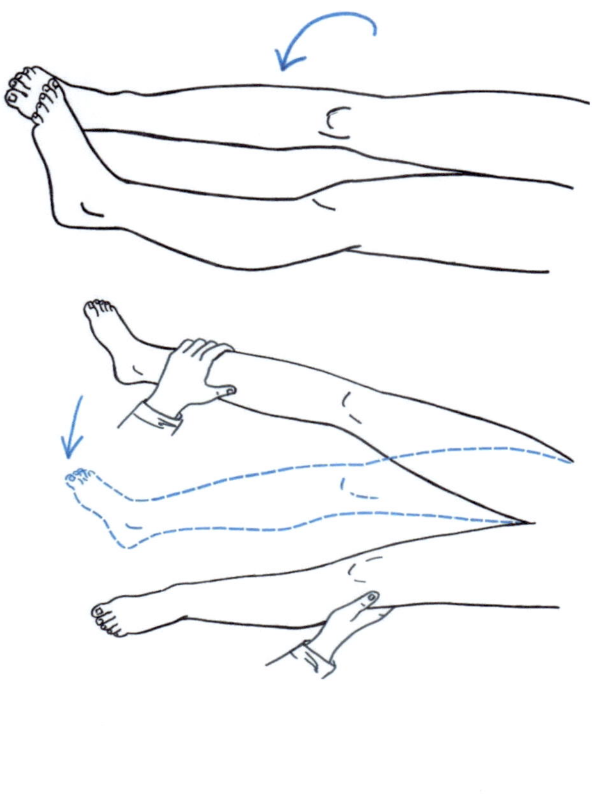

Fig. 18.36 Lesion of the superior gluteal nerve—clinical symptoms (illustrated by Ms. Anna Francová)

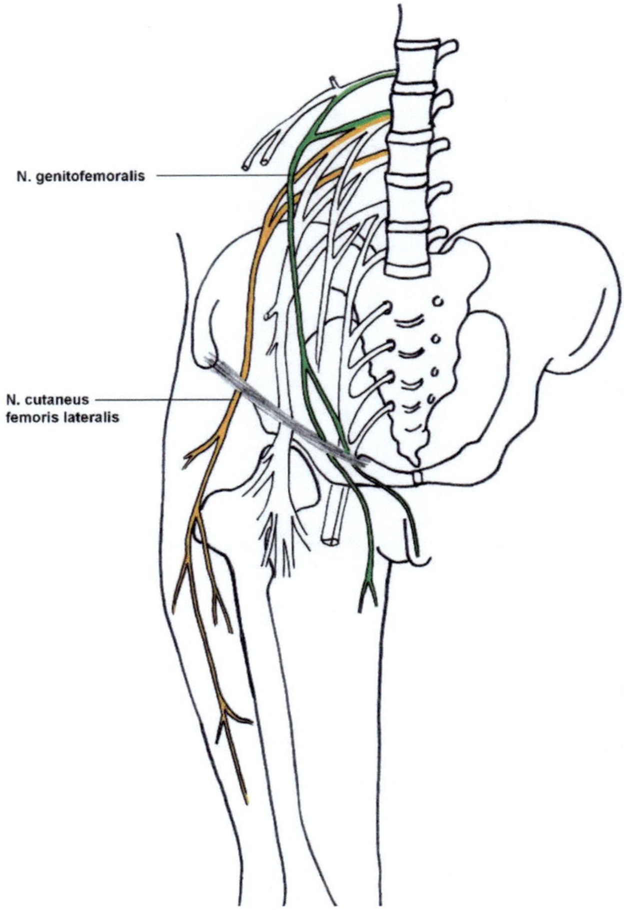

Fig. 18.37 Lateral cutaneous femoral nerve and genitofemoral nerve—formation (illustrated by Ms. Anna Francová)

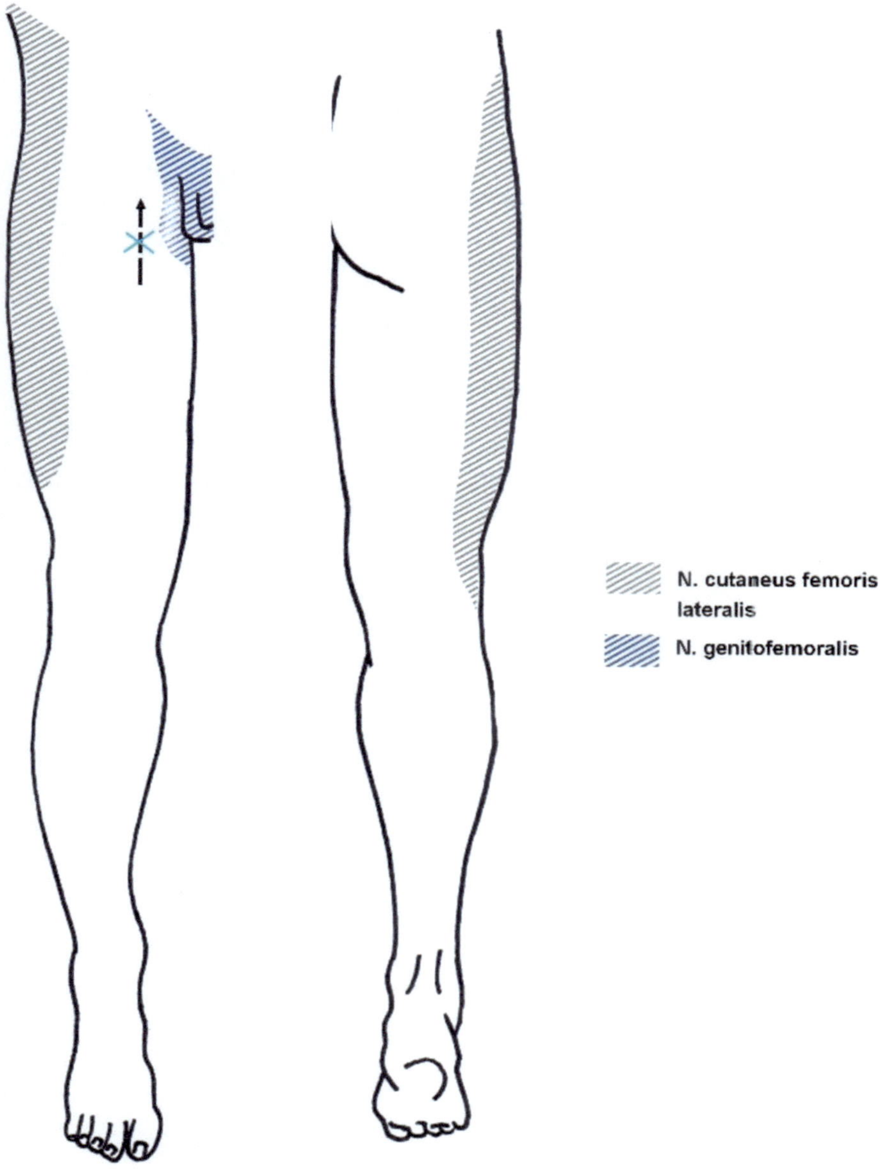

Fig. 18.38 Lesion of the lateral cutaneous femoral nerve and genitofemoral nerve—clinical symptoms (view from the back and front) (illustrated by Ms. Anna Francová)

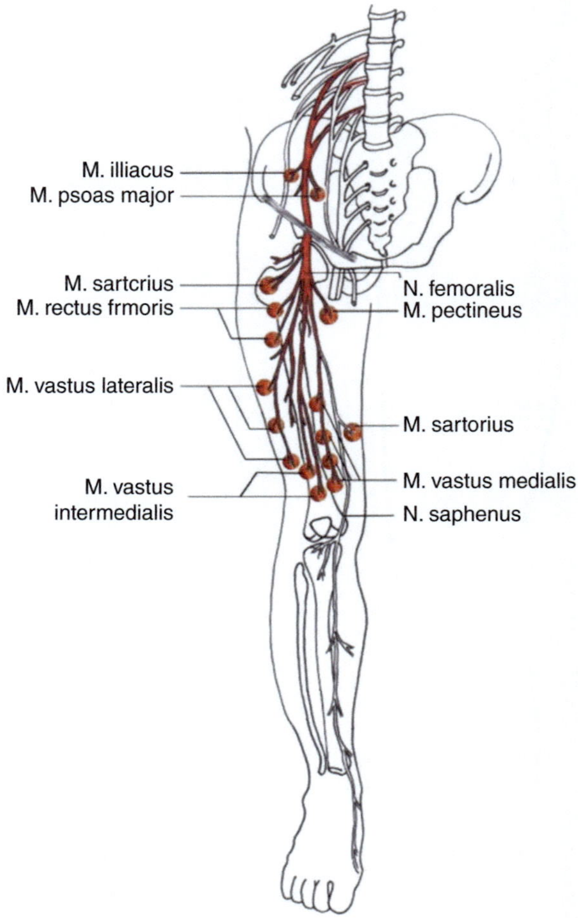

Fig. 18.39 Femoral nerve—innervation area (illustrated by Ms. Anna Francová)

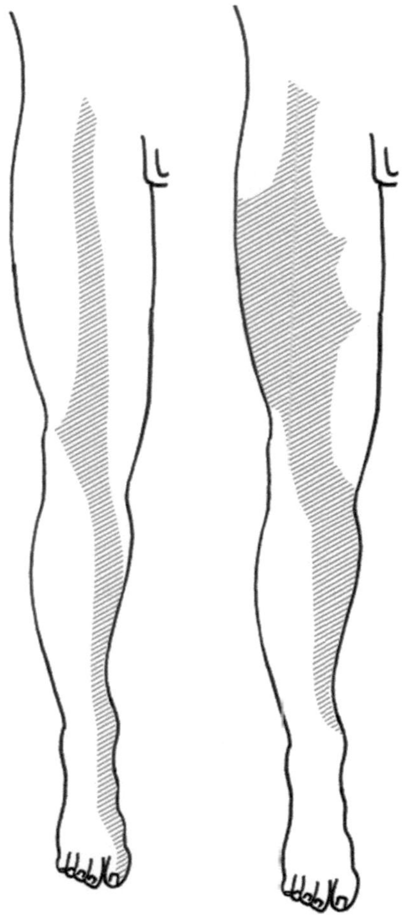

Fig. 18.40 Lesion of the femoral nerve—clinical examination and symptoms (illustrated by Ms. Anna Francová)

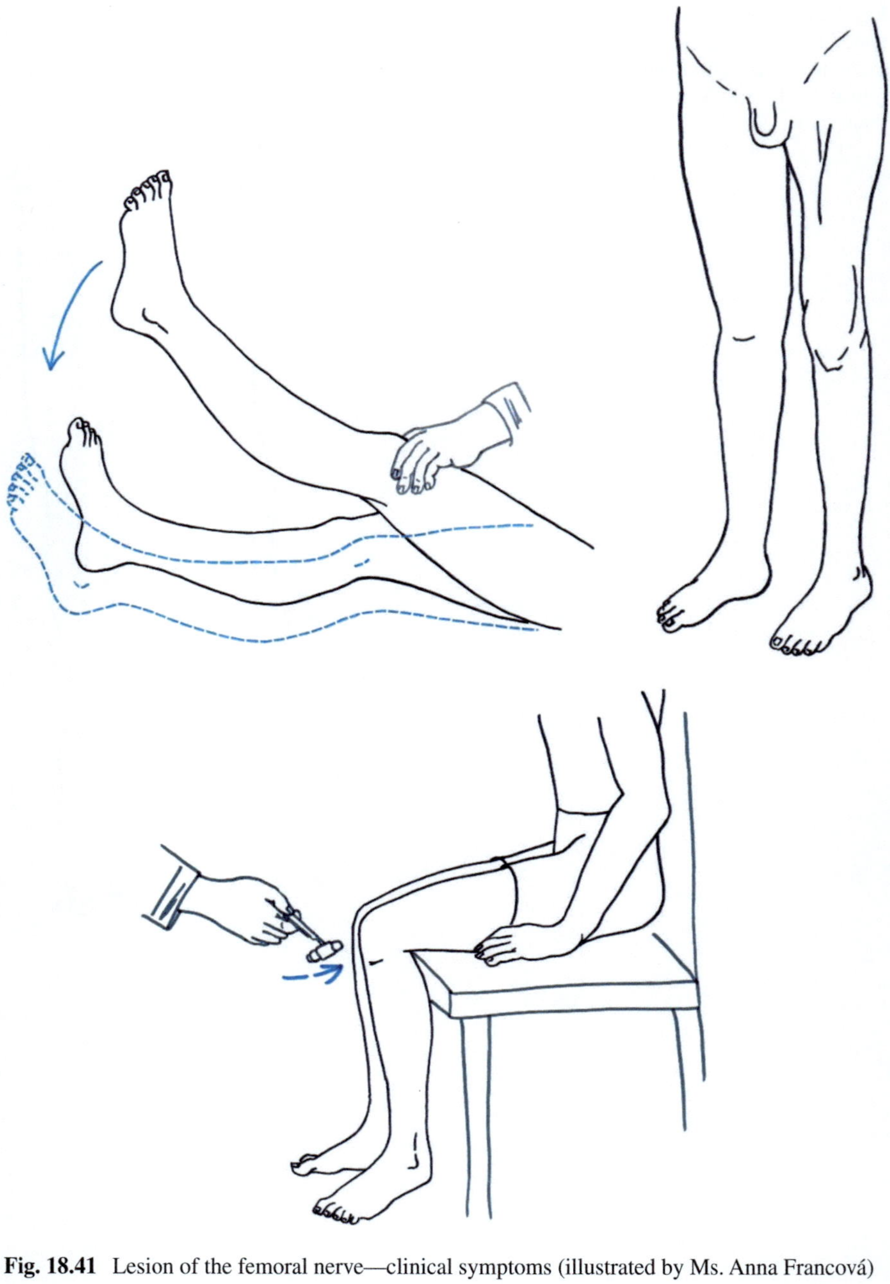

Fig. 18.41 Lesion of the femoral nerve—clinical symptoms (illustrated by Ms. Anna Francová)

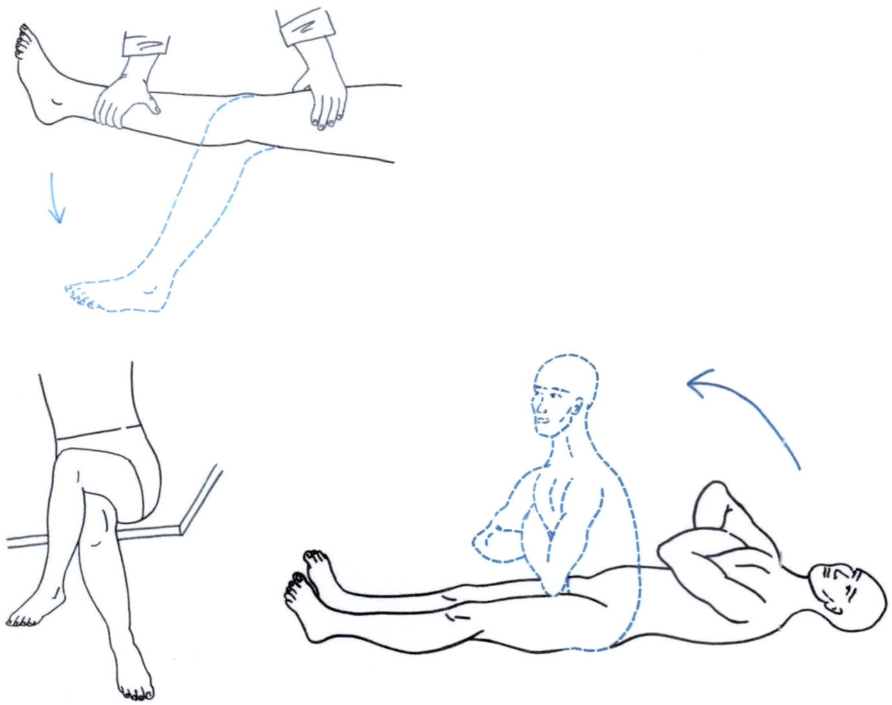

Fig. 18.42 Lesion of the femoral nerve—clinical symptoms (illustrated by Ms. Anna Francová)

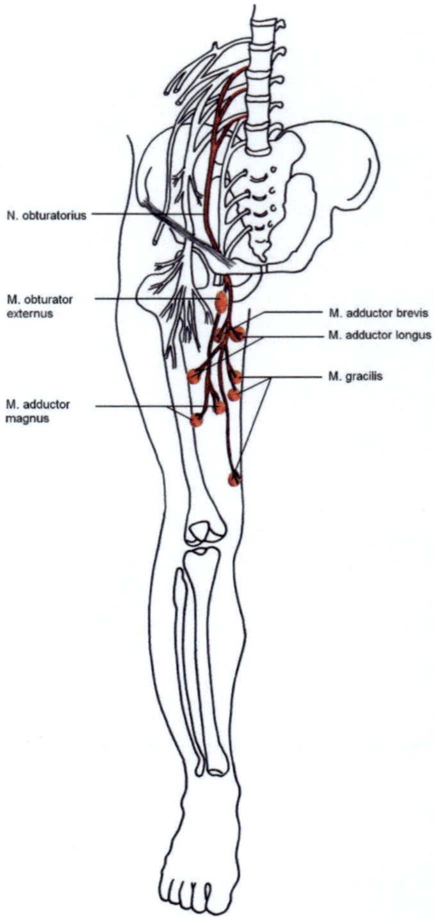

Fig. 18.43 Obturator nerve—innervation area (illustrated by Ms. Anna Francová)

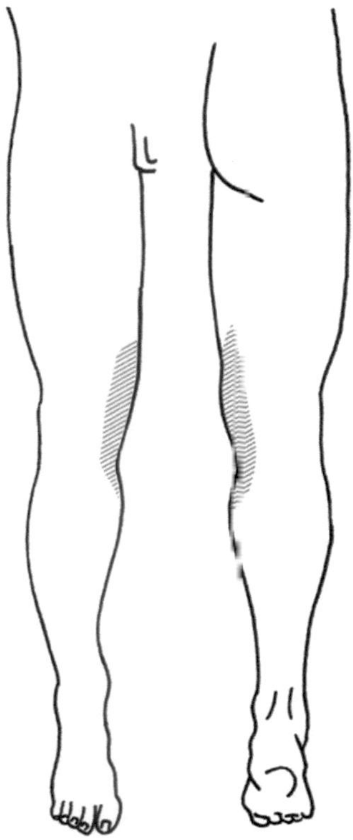

Fig. 18.44 Obturator nerve—clinical symptoms (illustrated by Ms. Anna Francová)

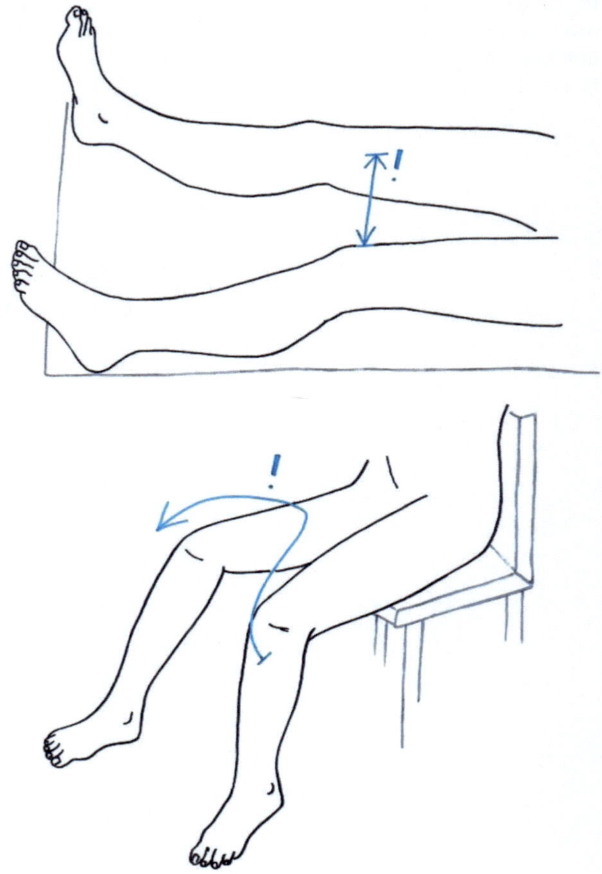

Fig. 18.45 Obturator nerve—clinical symptoms (illustrated by Ms. Anna Francová)

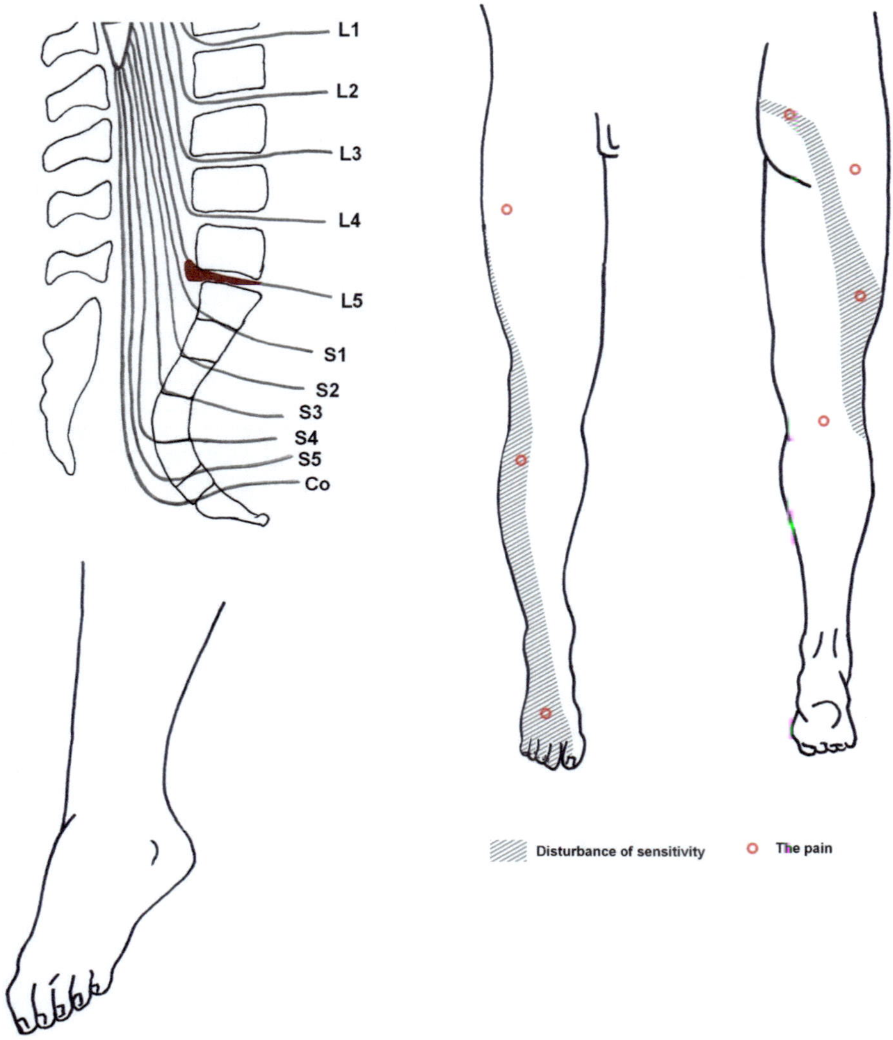

Fig. 18.46 Lesion of the root L5—clinical symptoms (illustrated by Ms. Anna Francová)

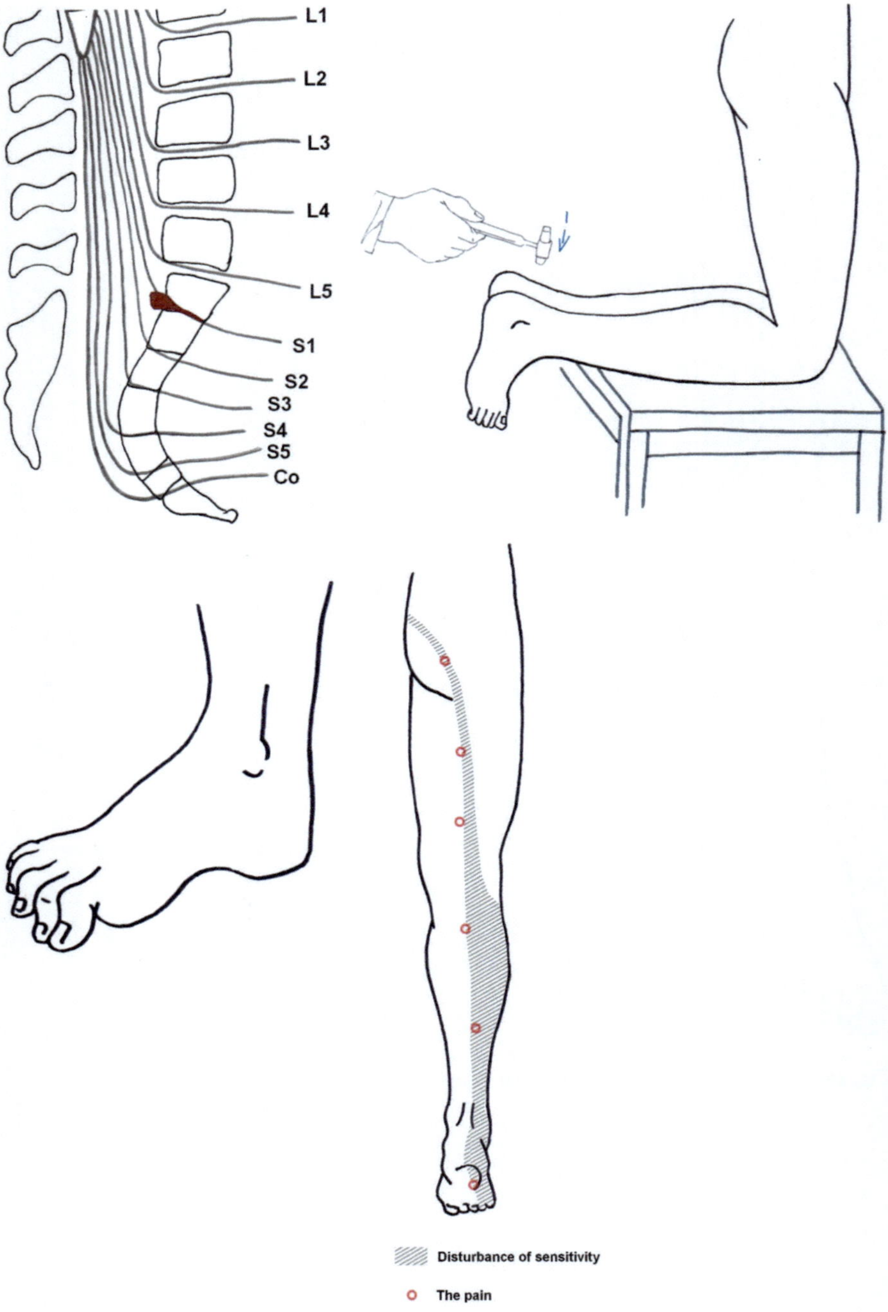

Fig. 18.47 Lesion of the root S1—clinical symptoms (illustrated by Ms. Anna Francová)

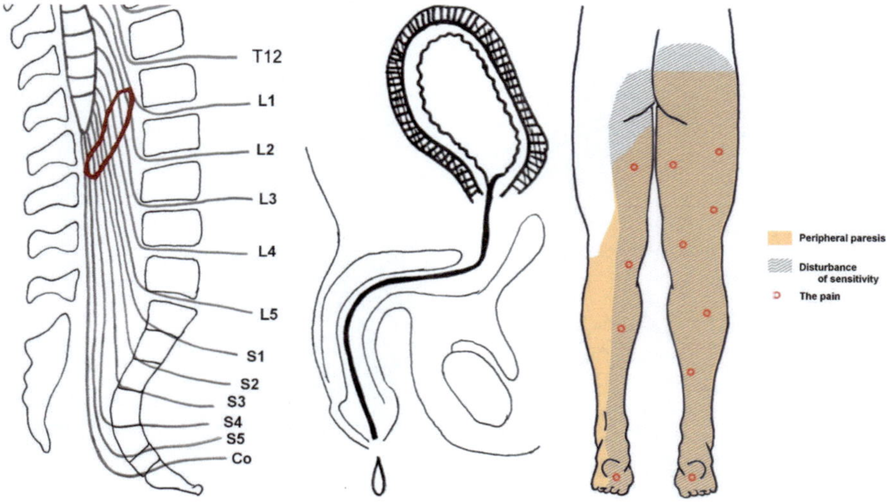

Fig. 18.48 Cauda equina lesions—clinical symptoms (illustrated by Ms. Anna Francová)

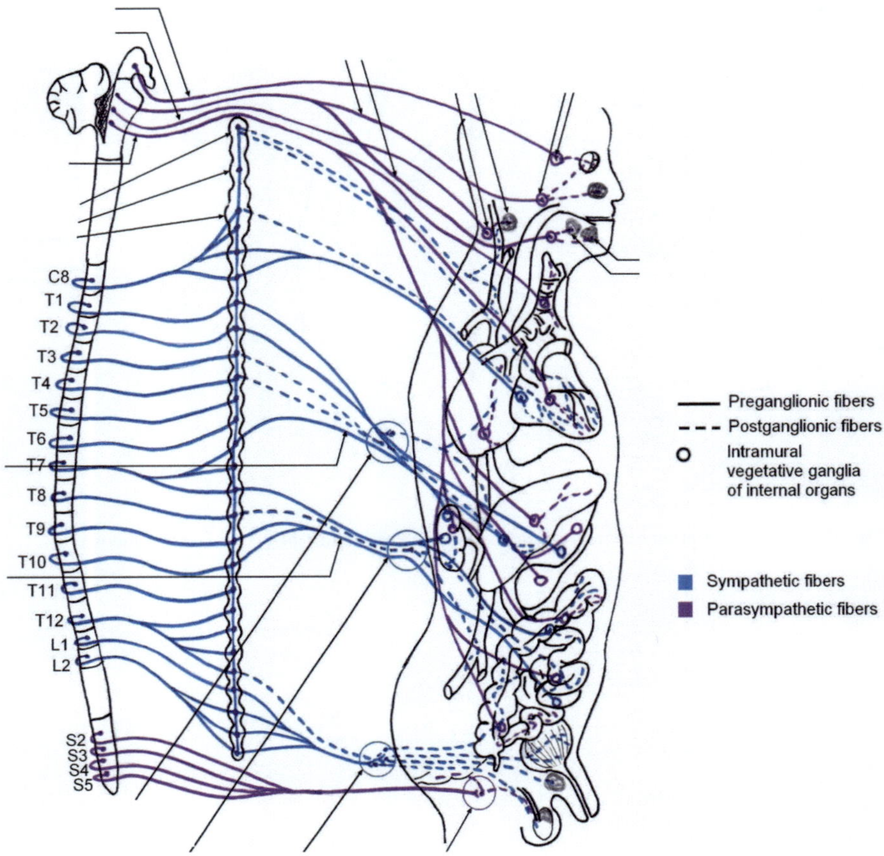

Fig. 18.49 Segmental level of the autonomic nervous system and sympathetic and parasympathetic innervation (illustrated by Ms. Anna Francová)

Bibliography

Aliotta RE, Jacob DD, Drake RL, Gurunian L, Gurunian R. Brachial artery and basilic/cephalic veins. Recipient vessels in reconstructive microsurgery: anatomy and technical considerations, 2021 141–148.

Arey LB. Development anatomy. Philadelphia and London: W.B. Saunders Company; 1940.

Baader B, Herrmann M. Topography of the pelvic autonomic nervous system and its potential impact on surgical intervention in the pelvis. Clin Anat. 2003;16(2):119–30.

Balik V, Šulla I. Autonomic dysreflexia following spinal cord injury. Asian J Neurosurg. 2022;17(2):165–72.

Bergman RA, Thompson SA, Afifi AK, Saddeh FA. Compendium of human anatomical variations. Urban and Schwarzenburg. Baltimore, 1988; s. 138–9.

Bergman RA, Afifi KA, Miyauchi R. Illustrated encyclopedia of human anatomic variation. Opus III: nervous system. 2015. Available online: https://www.anatomyatlases.org/AnatomicVariants/NervousSystem/Introduction.shtml (Accessed 23 Dec 2022).

Berthelot JM, Douane F, Ploteau S, Le Goff B, Darrieutort-Laffite C. Venous congestion as a central mechanism of radiculopathies. Joint Bone Spine. 2022;89(2):105291.

Cahill DR, Leonard RJ. Missteps and masquerade in American medical academe: clinical anatomists call for action. Clin Anat. 1999;12(3):220–2.

Chotigavanich C, Sawangnatra S. Anomalies of the lumbosacral nerve roots. An anatomic investigation. Clin Orthop Relat Res. 1992;278:46–50.

Coquet T, Lefranc M, Chenin L, Foulon P, Havet É, Peltier J. Unilateral duplicated abducens nerve coursing through both the sphenopetroclival venous gulf and cavernous sinus: a case report. Surg Radiol Anat. 2018;40(7):835–40. Erratum in: Surg Radiol Anat. 2018; 40 (11): 1327

Da Ros V, Picchi E, Ferrazzoli V, Schirinzi T, Sabuzi F, Grillo P, et al. Spinal vascular lesions: anatomy, imaging techniques and treatment. Eur J Radiol Open. 2021;8:100369.

Edwards LF, Baker RC. Variations in the formation of the splanchnic nerves in man. Anat Rec. 1940;77(3):335–42.

Erbil KM, Onderoğlu S, Başar R. Unusual branching in lumbar plexus: case report. Folia Morphol (Warsz). 1998;57(4):377–81.

Feigl GC, Schmid M, Zahn PK, González CAA, Litz RJ. The posterior femoral cutaneous nerve contributes significantly to sensory innervation of the lower leg: an anatomical investigation. Br J Anaesth. 2020;124(3):308–13.

Fye WB. Profiles in cardiology: William Osler. Clin Cardiol. 1988;11(5):356–8.

Gandhi KR, Verma VK, Chavan SK, Joshi SD, Joshi SS. The morphology of lumbar sympathetic trunk in humans: a cadaveric study. Folia Morphol (Warsz). 2013;72(3):217–22.

Z. Haviarová et al., *Peripheral Nervous System*,
https://doi.org/10.1007/978-3-031-73744-2

Haninec P, Kaiser R. Operační léčba poranění plexus brachialis. Č Sl Neurol Neurochir. 2011;74/107(5):619–30.

Hauck EF, Wittkowski W, Bothe HW. Intradural microanatomy of the nerve roots S1-S5 at their origin from the conus medullaris. J Neurosurg Spine. 2008;9(2):207–12.

Holmes LB. Current concepts in genetics. Congenital malformations. N Engl J Med. 1976;295(4):204–7.

Hulín I et al. Patofyziológia. 1998, Faber, 1141 s.

Ipsalali HO, Ciftci AC, Kilic D, Sendemir G, Seyhan S, Kaya I, Ortug G. Variations of the 6th cranial nerve (nervus abducens) in the petroclival region: a microsurgical study. Morphologie. 2019;103(341 Pt 2):103–9.

Iszi Y, Gürkncar D, Ozan H, Gönül E. The morphological aspects of lumbar plexus and roots. An anatomical study. Turk Neurosurg. 2005;15(2):87–92.

Joo W, Yoshioka F, Funaki T, Rhoton JR. Microsurgical anatomy of the abducens nerve. Clin Anat. 2012;25(8):1030–42.

Kachlík D, Varga I, Báča V, Musil V. Variant anatomy and its terminology. Medicina (Kaunas). 2020;56(12):713.

Kahle W, Frotscher M. Color atlas and textbook of human anatomy. Volume 3: nervous system and sensory organs. 5th ed. Stuttgart: Thieme Verlag; 2002.

Kapeller K. Štruktúra autonómneho nervového vlákna. Bratislava, Veda. 1979, 160 s.

Karemaker JM. An introduction into autonomic nervous function. Physiol Meas. 2017;38(5):R89–R118.

Lanz T, Wachsmuth W. Kopf: Űbergeordnete systeme, Teil A. Formentwiclung des Kopfes. Teil B. Gehirn- und Augenschädel. Praktische Anatomie, Springer-Verlag. Sonder Ausgabe. 2004.

Lippert H, Pabst R. Arterial variations in man classification and frequency. München: J.F. Bergman Verlag; 1985.

Loukas M, Klaassen Z, Merbs W, Tubbs RS, Gielecki J, Zurada A. A review of the thoracic splanchnic nerves and celiac ganglia. Clin Anat. 2010;23(5):512–22.

Lovásová K, Šulla IJ, Boleková A, Šulla I, Kluchová D. Anatomical study of the roots of cranial parasympathetic ganglia: a contribution to medical education. Ann Anat. 2013;195(3):205–11.

Marden PM, Smith DW, McDonald MJ. Congenital anomalies in the newborn infant, including minor variations. J Pediatr. 1964;64:357–71.

Moore KL. Clinically oriented anatomy. 2nd ed. Baltimore: Williams & Wilkins; 1985. p. 626–793.

Moore KL, Dalley AL. Clinically oriented anatomy II. 5th ed. Baltimore, MD: Williams; 2006. p. 321.

Mullins BM, Kelsall N. Anatomy of the lumbar and sacral plexuses and lower limb peripheral neuropathies. Surgery (Oxford). 2023;41(4):193–9.

Nightingale TE, Mehnert U, Kessler TM, Krassioukov AV. Autonomous nervous system dysfunction. Oxford Textbook of Neurorehabilitation; 2020. p. 111.

Obersteiner H, Redlich E. Uber wesen und Patogenese der Tabischen Hinterstrangs Degeneration. ARB Neurol Inst Univ Wien. 1894;1-3:158–72.

O'Rahilly R, Müller F, Meyer DB. The human vertebral column at the end of the embryonic period proper. 4. The sacrococcygeal region. J Anat. 1990;168:95–111.

Pernkopf E. Atlas of topographical and applied human anatomy, Vol. 2: thorax and extremities, 2nd revised ed. Philadelphia, PA: W.B. Saunders Company; 1989. p. 1–308.

Rouviére H, Delmas A. Anatomie humaine. Descriptive, Topographique et Fonctionelle. 15th ed. Paris: Masson; 2002. p. 1–784. ISBN 9782294003929

Ruskell GL. Distribution of pterygopalatine ganglion efferents to the lacrimal gland in man. Exp Eye Res. 2004;78(3):329–35.

Sawyer FK, Stefanik JJ, Lufler RS. The branching and innervation pattern of the radial nerve in the forearm: clarifying the literature and understanding variations and their clinical implications. Diagnostics. 2020;10(6):366.

Shiozawa T, Herlan S, Wagner HJ, Küppers E. Surgical prosection in a traditional anatomical curriculum-Tübingens' Sectio chirurgica. Ann Anat. 2010;192(6):349–54.

Shoja MM, Tubbs RS. Augusta Déjerine-Klumpke: the first female neuroanatomist. Clin Anat. 2007;20:585–7. https://doi.org/10.1002/ca.20474.

Siéssere S, Vitti M, Sousa LG, Semprini M, Iyomasa MM, Regalo SC. Anatomic variation of cranial parasympathetic ganglia. Braz Oral Res. 2008;22(2):101–5.

Solmaz B, Tatarlı N, Ceylan D, Keleş E, Çavdar S. Intradural communication between dorsal rootlets of spinal nerves: their clinical significance. Acta Neurochir. 2015;157(6):1069–76. discussion 1076

Šteňová J, Kubíková E, Šteňo J. Topografické anatomické vzťahy chrbtice, miechy a miechových nervov, význam pre klinickú prax. Neurol pre prax. 2009;10(4):205–8.

Stevenson RE, Hall JG. Terminology, Vol. 1. In: Stevenson RE, Hall JG and Goodman RM (eds.). Human malformations and related anomalies. Oxford University Press, London. 1993, 21–30.

Šulla JI, Lukáč I, Šulla I. Syndroma cauda equinae discogenes. Košice: Univerzita Pavla Jozefa Šafárika; 2009. ISBN 978-80-7097-769-9

Šulla I, Balik V, Horňák S, Ledecký V. Cauda equina syndrome in dogs—review. Acta Vet Brno. 2018;87(4):321–33.

Swell RS. Clinical anatomy by regions. 7th ed. Baltimore: Livingstone; 2004. p. 991.

Takahashi Y, Sipp D, Enomoto H. Tissue interactions in neural crest cell development and disease. Science. 2013;341(6148):860–3.

Thakker MM, Huang J, Possin DE, Ahmadi AJ, Mudumbai R, Orcutt JC, Tarbet KJ, Sires BS. Human orbital sympathetic nerve pathways. Ophthalmic Plast Reconstr Surg. 2008;24(5):360–6.

Traynelis VC, Malone HR, Smith ZA, et al. Rare complications of cervical spine surgery: Horner's syndrome. Global Spine J. 2017;7(1_suppl):103S–8S. https://doi.org/10.1177/2192568216688184.

Tubbs RS, Custis JW, Salter EG, Sheetz J, Zehren SJ, Oakes WJ. Landmarks for the greater petrosal nerve. Clin Anat. 2005;18(3):210–4.

Tubbs RS, El-Zammar D, Loukas M, Cömert A, Cohen-Gadol AA. Intradural cervical root adjacent interconnections in the normal, prefixed, and postfixed brachial plexus. J Neurosurg Spine. 2009a;11(4):413–6.

Tubbs RS, Menendez J, Loukas M, Shoja MM, Shokouhi G, Salter EG, Cohen-Gadol A. The petrosal nerves: anatomy, pathology, and surgical considerations. Clin Anat. 2009b;22(5):537–44.

Tubbs RS, Shoja MM, Loukas M, editors. Bergman's comprehensive encyclopedia of human anatomic variation. Hoboken, NJ: John Wiley & Sons; 2016.

Urbanowitz Z. Connections between the lumbal and sacral plexus in man. Folia Morphol (Warsz). 1981;40(3):271–9.

Ward EM, Rorie DK, Nauss LA, Bahn RC. The celiac ganglia in man: normal anatomic variations. Anesth Analg. 1979;58(6):461–5.

Webber RH. Some variations in the lumbar plexus of nerves in man. Acta Anat (Basel). 1961;44:336–45.

Wiliams PL. Nervous system in Gray's anatomy. 38th ed. New York: Churchill Livingstone; 1995. p. 1267–72.

Yang HJ, Gil YC, Lee WJ, Kim TJ, Lee HY. Anatomy of thoracic splanchnic nerves for surgical resection. Clin Anat. 2008;21(2):171–7.

Zhang Y, Liu H, Liu EZ, Lin YZ, Zhao SG, Jing GH. Microsurgical anatomy of the ocular motor nerves. Surg Radiol Anat. 2010;32(7):623–8.

Zvěřina E, Stejskal L. Poranění periférních nervů. Praha: Avicenum; 1979. p. 303.

Zvěřina E, Chovanec M, Betka J. Rekonštrukční operace lícního nervu v zadní jáme a v mostovomozečkového koutu. In: Vachata P., Sameš M. et al. Lícní nerv. Mladá Fronta 2016. pp.141–159. ISBN 978-80-204-3252-0.

MIX
Papier aus verantwortungsvollen Quellen
Paper from responsible sources
FSC® C105338

If you have any concerns about our products,
you can contact us on
ProductSafety@springernature.com

In case Publisher is established outside the EU,
the EU authorized representative is:
Springer Nature Customer Service Center GmbH
Europaplatz 3, 69115 Heidelberg, Germany

Printed by Libri Plureos GmbH
in Hamburg, Germany